PRAISE

With *Mirth* and Laughter

"From her own encounter and suffering with breast cancer, Dr. Thompson fashions a heartfelt, sharply-observed account of how her life changed for the better, and better doctoring. Her expertise in medicine is stretched to understand how to be a patient/doctor, and then movingly extends to her journey to learn and practice good connection with other patients. She's a beacon to her practice, her students, and her family. The book is a primer on empathy between doctor and patient. A vibrant, touching, honest work."

—Samuel Shem, M.D., Professor of Medicine at NYU Medical School, author of *The House of God* and the upcoming sequel, *Man's 4th Best Hospital*

"This is a book in two conjoined parts by the author, a doctor, whose first response to the discovery of her breast cancer was shock, confusion, and fear. Oddly enough, that tumor discovery is the event (for a gifted mind and spirit such as hers) that allows her to provide the very best attention to her care, for both her patients and her teaching of younger doctors and medical students. She is, by her experience, the deeply understanding physician who seeks, as is evidenced during the second part of her story, to augment care of her patients by the most important tool any doctor can have: empathy. Empathy is not sympathy, nor 'niceness', nor even clinical excellence. It is, rather, the knowledge that whatever the patient is suffering can be recognized in a short sentence: 'It could be me' because, in fact, it was her. This book is well worth reading, not just for doctors and patients, but for all who care about the suffering of others."

—Faith Fitzgerald, M.D., MACP, Professor of Medicine at UC-Davis and frequent contributor to *On Being a Doctor*, Annals of Internal Medicine

PRAISE

With Mirth and Laughter

"How delightful it was for me, years after my breast cancer diagnosis, to read the words of a physician who walked the same path. Dr. Thompson's ability to successfully choreograph her profession, family, and provide self-care was beautifully displayed in *With Mirth and Laughter.*

As an author, I admire Dr. Thompson's resolve and fervency to pen her experiences and touch the world in ways only she could. As a pastor, I especially applaud her open and bold expressions of faith in God that carried her through this challenge and still does to this day.

For any patient, *With Mirth and Laughter* presents an opportunity to learn the arduous task of being a physician while wrestling with cancer. It was a reminder for me to lend compassion and patience in return to the health care professionals who so sincerely care, and who have their own stories. I highly recommend this read to all people whose world has been interrupted by cancer. You will be enlightened, encouraged and comforted."

—Teresa E. Nelson, breast cancer survivor, Pastor of Tibbetts Brook Chapel and author of *Tender Mercies for Tough Moments*

To Macy—

With *Mirth* and Laughter

HEATHER THOMPSON BUUM, M.D.

*Thank you for the support!
—Heather*

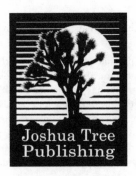

Joshua Tree
Publishing

• Chicago •

With *Mirth* and Laughter
HEATHER THOMPSON BUUM, M.D.

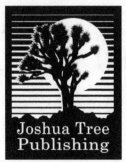

Joshua Tree
Publishing

Published by
Joshua Tree Publishing
• Chicago •
JoshuaTreePublishing.com

13-Digit ISBN: 978-1-941049-55-6

Front Cover Image Credit: © cienpiesnf

Cover Background Image Credit: © THesIMPLIFY

Bible verses are from unless noted: New International Version (NIV)
Holy Bible, New International Version®, NIV® Copyright ©1973, 1978, 1984, 2011 by Biblica, Inc.® Used by permission. All rights reserved worldwide.

New American Standard Bible (NASB)
Copyright © 1960, 1962, 1963, 1968, 1971, 1972, 1973, 1975, 1977, 1995 by The Lockman Foundation

Credits for previously published chapters are listed in Credits, page 214.

Disclaimer:

Printed in the United States of America

"With mirth and laughter, let old wrinkles come.
And let my liver heat with wine
than my heart cool with mortifying groans."
—William Shakespeare, *Merchant of Venice*

TABLE OF CONTENTS

Chapter 1

To Everything There
Is a Season

The harvest now is over, the summer days are gone.
—Mendelssohn's *Elijah*

Mid-August should feel lush and lazy, heavy with heat and humidity, the dog days of summer as they say. The local farmer's markets and neighborhood gardens bring forth their bounty: ripe and juicy tomatoes, plump and shining bell peppers, fragrant basil, melons that are heavy, taut, and emanating potent scents. The lakes have turned green with algae; a chartreuse slick of foam is floating on the south side of Lake Como. I watch it grow day by day on my morning run. Later, there is a bit of mist or fog in the cool morning air, and morning sunlight starts to appear long, low, and golden. The geese are flying overhead, honking, V-formation, announcing tentative plans to migrate to the nearby harvest fields.

The other side of August: a slight melancholy, a tension, a hint of sadness and of loss. Although September and October are glorious in Minnesota—crisp and sunny fall weather, low humidity, followed by an amazing display of colorful leaves—it is, to be sure, a harbinger of things to come. Fall is too short, too rapid of a descent into colder temperatures and the eventual onslaught of winter, including snow, sleet, snow plows, snow shoveling, ice, black ice, ice dams, below-zero wind-chill, school cancellations, or two-hour delayed start, followed by over an hour commute five miles into work through the snow, passing cars spun out into the ditch.

Despite my recent cancer diagnosis and constantly reminding myself that "every day is a gift, take it one day at a time, don't look too far ahead," I can't help but have these August melancholy moments, in part due to my children. Sam, almost twelve, entering sixth grade; Lydia, age nine, entering fourth. For both of them, I am getting bombarded with constant reminders about the pending start of the school year. The forms to be signed, the long list of school supplies to be purchased, the upcoming schedule changes for the middle school students—they actually start sending these things out end of *July*, causing undue stress. Sam and Lydia are not too thrilled about it either; soon will be gone the days of sleeping in, going for bike rides around the lake, or hanging out in the backyard with the neighbor kids. And although they enjoy school, their friends, their teachers, it's a rough transition, to say the least. I also do *not* appreciate our local Target store setting out school supplies right after the Fourth of July or my neighborhood Cub Foods stocking a Halloween candy display on *August 16!* Come on, people! We don't need these reminders when it's still eighty degrees and sunny and we should be reading a good book in a hammock or spending the day at the lake.

I am in such denial that I have not gone school shopping at all, either online or in person, nor done any preparation, such as the physicals or the form completion, when my family is invited to a pool party on a Sunday afternoon in August. This is being hosted at the home of a family whose two girls are each in both Sam's and Lydia's classes. Paul and I decide to join them. We're free that day; I respond with a yes via e-mail. Four families attend in total, all from our school, enjoying the warm summer afternoon, kids splashing in the pool, adults lounging poolside with great food and a nice glass of wine. But right away, every mom starts comparing notes. One asks, "Which store is most high yield for that long list of school supplies sent weeks ago? Is it Target? Walmart? Staples?" Another replies, "What about those red correcting pencils? So hard to find!" They ask me where I have gone, and with a nervous laugh, I say, "Gee, I must admit, I have not done anything yet." They smile politely, and although I do very much enjoy these women and their company and the adult conversation, these thoughts cross my mind: *Is this really all that important? Who cares?* After going through breast cancer treatment, including surgery, medication and physical therapy, it seems I really don't sweat the little things anymore. And I want to hold on to every precious moment of summer. I would almost rather go to the store the *very night before* the first day of school because then we don't have to stare at a pile of three-ring binders on the dining-room table for the coming weeks, reminding us all that the end is near. One woman comments, "Target is really picked over by now." I think, *Oh well, online shopping to the rescue.*

I'm trying not to sound negative or cynical, but sometimes I marvel at how much my perspective has changed. And I am not exactly sure, in this moment in time, if this is a good thing or a bad thing. I *should* pay attention, at some point, to things such as hot lunch order forms, right? But lately, I'm having a hard time with that. I would rather read a good book, listen to music, write, sing, go on a three-mile run or a bike ride, walk onto a golf course, or spend all Saturday afternoon in my kitchen, making pickled beets and homemade salsa. I'm finding no matter how much I try, I have a hard time motivating myself for anything other than what I might find truly enjoyable. I chastise myself constantly, thinking, *How selfish! Self-centered! When are you going to snap out of this!* On the other hand, later, I will read a post on Facebook, or a prayer request in our church bulletin, or an obituary in the local paper, some woman who has a new diagnosis of breast cancer, is now fighting metastatic breast cancer, or has succumbed to the disease. And at that point, I am right back to square one. I wonder, contemplate, and conclude—none of us really knows how much time we have left. And that includes me now.

Back at the pool party, I'm chatting with the same group of women, all in their mid- to late forties. They are discussing menopause or perimenopause and the difficult time they are having—the hot flashes, insomnia, fatigue. I am sitting there, half in the shade of a patio umbrella, half in the sun. It's not really that hot or humid; it's barely eighty degrees and a nice breeze, yet under my miniskirt, sweat is running down the back of my legs. It is dripping actually, making physical drops on the flagstone patio that is underneath my feet as I clutch the glass of Chardonnay and contemplate holding it up against my forehead. Inwardly, I think, *Try being on tamoxifen!* I am too warm, hot, and overheated. I feel feverish constantly, all the time, and not just in flashes. Although I do have these interesting "waves" of searing, burning sensations; they start in my lower abdomen, then generalize, then end with my face turning red as a beet. I have not slept past 5:00 a.m. in months. Since they know I am an MD, they ask my opinion on all this. "What do you think about taking bio-identical hormones? Does that help relieve symptoms?" Another asks about dietary interventions, such as soy milk, edamame. Someone mentions yam progesterone. We chat about this, but I am thinking to myself, *As a breast cancer survivor, I should avoid any and all hormonal manipulation like the plague even if it is deemed "natural" and/or "homeopathic."* That's what got me into trouble in the first place, after all, with a tumor that was strongly ER/PR positive. I just have to put up with a host of symptoms, these side effects, this new medical menopause, and endure, carry on. No yam progesterone for me.

Here's the other thing I find a bit unfair: I packed my swimsuit for this outing, and I'm totally overheated, and I just want to jump into that inviting pool and go for a nice dip, a swim, and cool-off. However, none of the other moms will don their suits—not sure if it is modesty or self-consciousness or what exactly. Later, all the dads somehow get the nerve to change into swim trunks and jump in, hairy backs, beer guts, and all. They splash around, throw balls to the kids, and float by on the inflatable rafts. Why is it that the men in our society seem to have none of these "issues"? I also think, I'm just a few months out from a right mastectomy, no reconstruction. If anyone should be body conscious, it should be me! Not these other moms who are all trim and fit, perfectly pedicured, and I am fairly certain can fill out their swim top with their own God-given bosoms. Gee, here I spent all that time sewing a disc-shaped foam pad into the right side of my red and white polka-dot one-piece, and now I don't even get to wear it.

Sigh. I'm back to this negative attitude again, which is so unlike me. I try to remind myself again of the many blessings

I've had over the past few months; I'm on tamoxifen, not *chemo*. I didn't need radiation; my lymph nodes were negative. I had a quick post-op recovery, back to work in two weeks. I had amazing medical care and support from friends, family members, church family, neighbors, and colleagues. I keep reminding myself what the alternatives could have been.

I also think I'm just in a bit of a funk, honestly, because Charlie and his family are in Sun Valley, Idaho, for three weeks. I have come to realize I am missing my colleague and mentor, now lunch companion, coffee mate, sounding board. Before this diagnosis, the advice from Charlie was mostly career-related; navigating promotion and tenure, publishing an article, submitting grants, and the like. Lately, it's that, but it's also sharing advice, observations, perspectives, on anything and everything, on life itself. What it's like to have to deal with a new cancer diagnosis. Adjusting to activity restrictions after surgery. How physical issues can change personal relationships, friendships, intimacy, and so on. Tolerating side effects from a new drug or from radiation treatment. Wondering, always a bit fearful about the next steps, the next scan or imaging study, the lab test, and other follow-ups that must occur. These conversations have been immensely helpful to me in ways I never thought possible.

In fact, after he retired in 2016, I had the sinking sensation that I might not see him all that often . . . or maybe ever again. At a very fit and functional seventy-seven, I reasoned he and his wife, Gay, will want to travel extensively, especially while they are both still in good health. Also, his retirement party, hosted at the governor's mansion on Summit, was a Friday evening end of February. Unfortunately, the same night, my son Sam was also playing in a basketball tournament. I felt obligated to attend Sam's game instead and cheer him on. They got whomped, absolutely crushed by a local Catholic school, kids that I swear were over six feet tall in fifth grade. Too bad I had to miss Charlie's retirement party for *that*.

But later, he comes out of retirement, working on a part time basis; still filling in for resident clinic and small groups and occasionally adding clinic sessions of his own. And then irony of ironies, two months into this and we would have the extreme bonding experience of both being diagnosed with cancer, different types, but operated on by the same surgeon just weeks apart while covering each other's resident clinic and teaching responsibilities during the post-op recovery period. Since then, as a result of all this, it's become more than just a mentoring relationship; it's almost like a father-daughter relationship. It's unique, perhaps the first time in my life that I've felt this comfortable confiding in someone about so many different things; I appreciate the support on multiple levels. And looking back, there is definitely a reason for all this happening, a sense that this was meant to be, too many "coincidences" to believe this was all driven by chance.

So while Charlie and Gay and their children and grandkids enjoy Sun Valley, with the pristine weather, low humidity, lack of mosquitoes, and so on, I must attempt to enjoy this pool party. Here we are—it's a perfect afternoon, great company, fabulous food, and we're sitting in a side yard overlooking Lake of the Isles in Minneapolis, taking in a beautiful view. And I do start to enjoy myself very much honestly after I disband my negative thoughts and disrupt my inner pity party about being on tamoxifen. It doesn't take much effort actually; in the worldly sense, I tend to be a rather positive person, an optimist—glass is always half full. I try to find the humor in everything; laughter is, indeed, the best medicine. In the spiritual realm, I believe God is in control and has a plan, and I simply have to trust and follow along. This may sound overly simplistic, but for me, it's the only way to live.

There is a verse from Ecclesiastes: "To everything there is a season, a time for every purpose under Heaven." This season, this time, late summer, should perhaps be the most cherished of all, given the harsh Minnesota winter that is soon to follow. I get up from the patio chair, stretch my legs a bit, and walk over to the steps leading down to the water. I could at least dip my feet in; that truly goes a long way to lower my inner thermostat, which is so entirely out of whack right now. I get out my phone, careful not to drop it in the water, and take a few pictures: Lydia flashing a big grin, her eyes smiling behind the swim goggles, floating on a noodle next to the other girls. Sam leaping off the stone wall on the east side of the pool, catching a nerf ball thrown to him from below and landing in the deep end. The entire drill actually appears somewhat unsafe but so much fun I decide to let it go. I then climb back up the stairs and walk over to the pool house behind this structure. In the shade of the tall oaks, I snap a photo of Paul and three other dads on the shuffleboard court.

I put away the phone and head over to sample the wood-fired pizzas now coming out of the stone fireplace on the back patio. Wow, the "caramelized onion and blue cheese" version is fantastic. If there is one positive aspect of a cancer diagnosis, it's having a new appreciation for the simple pleasures in life, great food definitely being one of them. Overall, it has been a lovely afternoon, and I am once again reminded of how good it is to be surrounded by family, friends, and yes, sunshine and eighty degrees even if it is only for a few more weeks. I will try to keep this in mind next time I am weathering another wave of an extreme hot flash. Or even better, with my new reset thermostat, maybe a fifteen-degree day in January will feel actually feel balmy to me! Another positive note!

Also from Ecclesiastes: "Then I commended mirth, because a man hath no better thing under the sun, than to eat, and to drink, and to be merry; for that shall abide with him all the days of his life."

Amen to that.

Chapter 2

BACK TO TEACHING

Into the great wide open,
Under them skies of blue . . .
—Tom Petty

B y midsummer, my work schedule had already shifted back into high gear. Mere weeks after surgery, and I'm back in clinic full-time. Soon I will have my first week of inpatient attending, and I also resume small-group teaching for the Essentials of Clinical Medicine course. The purpose of this small group, 10:00 a.m. to noon every Wednesday, is to have six to eight students each present a patient, a full history and physical, to prepare them for patient presentations on clinical rotations in the third and fourth year. The course runs for eight weeks, so I get to know the group of students fairly well. Since they have not yet experienced all of first- and second-year teaching, my role is often to explain to them how to put symptoms and/or physical exam findings into a clinical context—such as why you really need to ask about cough or chest pain in a patient with sudden onset shortness of breath, or how it is important to look for the presence or absence of ascites in a patient with suspected liver disease.

Often, I find myself taking creative license, asking the group, "Well, what *would* you expect to find on physical exam, or have asked during the history?" Because so many times, unfortunately, they are assigned a patient on the wards who is completely demented or near comatose, or the patient was suddenly whisked off to radiology and they never had a chance to even attempt the physical exam. It would be a tough rotation for an early first- or second-year student. I have taken to giving them very short one- to two-page handouts, a summary on such topics as atrial fibrillation, GI bleeding, pneumonia—common inpatient admitting problems. They contain the bare minimum: "Here's what you really need to know in order to evaluate a patient with this. You'll learn much more detail in the second-year pathophysiology courses, just wait." The students seem to really appreciate the short handouts and the practical approach.

At any rate, the two weeks I had off after surgery, the students were on hiatus; and then another two weeks after, Charlie covered for me. I was very grateful to have this extra help; his willingness to jump in as small-group facilitator was incredibly helpful to me. Not many colleagues would have felt comfortable doing that, but Charlie had also been assigned his own ECM small group in the past; he knew the format very well. And I secretly suspect he really enjoyed being back in the teaching role. In some ways, there is no such thing as a retired academic physician, believe me.

Reporting to my first small-group session, I am back after being gone for four weeks in total. Before, when I told the students I was going to be out and the good Dr. Moldow was my substitute teacher, I felt I had to offer some explanation. I mentioned I was having surgery but left out the details, reassuring them I should be returning to finish the course, God willing and the creek don't rise. Then I think Charlie may have alluded to the fact that we were both becoming patients in our own system when he led the small-group discussion. Whatever the case may be, when I walk into the room, a small conference room on the sixth floor of Mayo, I sense something. I see six pairs of rather wide eyes staring at me with some concern, a tiny bit of fear, wondering what to say, if they dare ask anything.

"Welcome back!" one says. "I hope the surgery went well!" says another. I sit down and again contemplate, *How much do I really volunteer here?* I am having a hard time lately with the concept of TMI (too much information) versus what might actually be of benefit to some people in some small way. The last time I thought TMI, though, was when one of our staff physicians was talking about Viagra in the collaboration zone. Mine seems rather tame, honestly, by comparison.

I decide to start with humor! Of course! My go-to as of late. I tell them, "It's been a long time since I was a third-year medical student scrubbing into the operating rooms on the third floor of that building, and really, it hasn't changed a bit. It looks exactly the same. And my recent experience was actually far more pleasant than holding retractors for hours on end or getting rapped on the knuckles with a hemostat." They laugh. For now, I leave out the details of exactly what my operation was for, but it's a really good icebreaker. They start to open up.

"I've had brain surgery just last winter," blurts out a lovely young woman to my left. I had been wondering why her medical school photo on my grading sheet looks so different from her appearance now; it's the fact that she had long, wavy golden-brown hair in that photo and at this moment in time her hair is extremely short as if her head has been shaved. It is growing back in, but a bit uneven. It must have been about as long as Sinéad O'Connor in "Nothing Compares 2U." After hearing this, now I realize why. And that's pretty compelling. A young Asian man across the table from her says, "I had to have knee surgery in college." It's then that I think, *Hey, I have touched a nerve. And maybe in a good way.*

We spent the next few minutes not presenting patients but talking about what it is like being a patient who is also a part of the health-care system. Even a first-year medical student knows something, quite a bit actually, and that will give them a bit of perspective, even a bit of pause when we talk about things such as medical errors, operating on the wrong side of the body, and so on. These students have also just learned about sterile technique, including gowning and gloving in a workshop presented by the OR nurses. We chat about the OR in general and the odd experience of waking up from anesthesia. The conversation then turns toward pain medication. One student asks, "Why is it that no matter what the operation or what the perceived level of pain may be, that's it always the same amount of tablets of whatever narcotic dispensed: thirty. Is this some sort of magic number?"

I laugh and say, "That is very true. I still have twenty-eight oxycodone left in my medicine cabinet. I have no idea what to do with them."

Next, a riveting debate on the rise of prescription opioid drug abuse and what we as doctors or future doctors should be doing about it. Several references are again made to Prince and the recent tragedy, a talented musician and local icon lost to an overdose. I am sitting back, taking this all in; the students themselves are completely leading the discussion. One young lady talks at length about her service-learning project that involves Narcan training—to be able to allow family, loved ones, and others in the general public to respond to a potential opioid overdose. She talks about the early findings in her work, the lessons learned. I keep casually looking at my phone for the time, thinking, *Gee, I'm supposed to be teaching them something about presenting H & Ps. How long do I let this go on?*

I interject, and I offer a perspective from my own clinical practice. "You simply must have a pain contract with any patient who is needing opioids for more than just a couple of weeks and also have a nurse who is willing to go to bat for you." I describe Tony's approach; he's the nurse for Dr. Langland and me, and once we have a patient sign a pain contract, he completely abides by it no matter what reason. It's even a little bit good cop, bad cop. He might chastise them at times, calling in too soon for a refill. He'll say, "Really? Do you want Dr. Thompson to lose her license, her DEA number? The Feds are monitoring this!" No early refills, no replacing lost or stolen prescriptions, patients must have urine tox screens for monitoring and even a new approach, random pill counts. He may call a patient, have them present that very same day with their prescription pain meds in hand, and count the pills left in the bottle. If they are selling them or giving them away to friends or family or abusing it themselves, then they will not have the correct number of pills to get through the end of the month, and that's it. No more pain meds from Dr. Thompson or Dr. Langland—game over. They will see you for routine physicals and other follow-up, but sorry, we will no longer refill the OxyContin, Vicodin, Percocet, and it's up to you to figure out the next steps. There are plenty of over-the-counter remedies to be found.

This probably sounds very harsh, but over the fifteen years I've been in practice, it's saved me from sticky situations a number of times. And on the flip slide, it allows me to be completely comfortable prescribing the *necessary* amount of pain medication to someone who really needs it—such as the elderly man I followed for years with not one but *two* metastatic cancers to the bones, both prostate and renal cell, coupled with terrible arthritis pain. He was on *huge* doses of Dilaudid (yes, prescribed by me) in addition to a fentanyl patch; and he always walked into my clinic, very dapper in his fedora hat, sport coat, and cane—awake and alert as can be and with almost no pain.

Unfortunately, I worry that the patients we "fire" will just present somewhere else in the system to someone who is not paying quite this much attention, and the cycle starts all over again. Still, I share this with the students, not to frighten them or get on a soapbox but to continually emphasize how a team approach to delivering health care—including a capable call center, a really strong RN, helpful pharmacists, even the DEA website that monitors opioid prescriptions—is needed to address these complicated issues.

It is now nearing 11:00 a.m., and we only have one hour left to get through our six patient presentations. It's been a really great discussion, though. Nearing the end of it, I do share how much more respect I have for our own University of Minnesota doctors, nurses, and staff, and a deeper appreciation for the amazing care that I did receive right here, next door. Finally, we get started. One of the case presentations that follow from the students involves an adult with cystic fibrosis. He is fifty-two years old. Even that important fact is probably lost on them. I interrupt, and I say, "It was our very own team of dedicated pulmonologists under Dr. Warren Warwick that made incredible progress in the past few decades in cystic fibrosis lung disease, including vest therapy, antibiotic regimens." Their important work is what increased the life expectancy of CF patients from early thirties at most to now middle age and hopefully beyond—another success story, something to be shared with these young doctors in training. They should feel proud of their home institution.

This has been a very good session, and looking around the table, I feel it's been inspiring to them as well. And all this as a result of my saying essentially, "Hi, I'm back. I just had surgery." I didn't even have to divulge much in the way of details or personal information. Certainly, I didn't feel any TMI moments. Reflecting back, I think this teaching session was another turning point for me. I am thinking, *That wasn't too hard. How else could I use my recent experiences for a greater good, not just for me as a doctor but for my students, internal medicine residents, and other learners?* I am mulling this over well after small group concluded while walking over to start clinic.

That same afternoon, my first patient at one o'clock is Laurie, a physician herself close to my age with a complex medical history. During my medical leave, she stopped by in person to talk with my nurse Tony and asked about me; she wanted to know if everything was okay. Today, she's early as usual, arriving at 12:15 p.m. for a 1:00 p.m. appointment. I ask my medical assistant to please room her; I'm there early as well. I'll skip lunch for now and eat later, taking a chance I might get a no-show or an easy pre-op or something.

Laurie is quickly ushered through the vital-signs area and into a room, and I knock and enter. I haven't even looked at her chart yet, but Tony has been giving me updates. She's sitting in the chair, viewing something on her phone. She has very curly, shoulder-length dark hair, friendly brown eyes, a slightly round face, and full cheeks. She's been struggling with her weight due to some of the medications she's been on for the autoimmune disease. She looks up and seems really happy to see me. I shake her hand, sit down, and again, try to start with humor.

"You need to welcome me to the physicians with cancer club." Her dark-brown eyes widen. I tell her, "I've been diagnosed with early-stage breast cancer, but by all appearances, I can almost say I'm a survivor already."

She breathes a sigh of relief and says, "I am a charter member of that club. It's a small but select group of very neurotic individuals."

We laugh, and I tell her now how much more appreciation I have for what she's been through the past several years—the waiting, the worrying, the anxiety produced by every minuscule finding on a CT scan. Now we've both been there, and she agrees, it's a crazy place to be. Of course, we go on to review everything that went on for her while I was out. Unfortunately, Laurie now has osteonecrosis of the right tibia, presumably due to long-term steroid use. *Ouch.* When I see one medication, one intervention, one seemingly minor surgery or procedure leading to another then another, including now a list of fairly serious side effects and complications from chronic medications—that's really tough, that's the very difficult part of the continuity of care. Wishing you could somehow turn back the clock and make a different decision or consider an alternative all those years ago.

Still, we have a good chat, reviewing potential treatment plans and options; we are still waiting on some follow-up results as well as getting a few subspecialists to weigh in on this new finding. I order some labs and place the appropriate referrals. I get up, and as I am about ready to leave, we both lean in for a hug. It's been very good to open up to her after all, and for what it's worth, I think we both feel better about it.

So in the very same calendar day, I have shared at least part of my story with a group of medical students, then a patient of mine; and each time, it is met with a very positive response. I am struck by this fact. I even think, *Isn't this the opposite of what we are taught in medical school?* That in order to maintain a professional working environment, we need boundaries. We are taught in general not to reveal too much about ourselves. We don't want to compromise the doctor-patient relationship or detract from the objectivity. However, in doing so, we may be missing opportunities to make real connections, to allow authenticity and vulnerability to permeate that relationship. It's quite possibly the ultimate expression of empathy—to convey we've been there. We understand what it's like to be a patient.

Later, I get an e-mail from Laurie. She's shared with me as an attachment, a poem that she wrote right after the renal cell carcinoma diagnosis. She submitted it to *Minnesota Monthly,* and it was published in 2015. I read through it, contemplate the meaning of it, and also recognize so many similar emotional responses to my situation.

Cancer

Even though you think you are prepared for anything,

No one is prepared for that word at any time, no matter who they are.

Instantly, you become a patient, who is just as scared as any other patient but who knows more than most other patients, which now is not a good thing.

All that knowledge becomes your worst enemy as you wait first for evaluations by specialists and then a confirmatory diagnosis.

While most patients are looking on the Internet for information, you are poring over the latest medical journals and physician websites for information on the possible type of cancer and the statistics about those cancers and this becomes the scariest part of all as you wait for treatment.

The tricks your mind starts to play on you.

You automatically assume the worst because physicians are taught to prepare patients.

You wonder and hope that you will be in the survival group.

You begin to pray for contained disease, no lymphatic invasion, and no metastatic disease or maybe a miracle or a benign tumor.

All the while, deep down in the pit of your stomach you think,

CANCER, I KNOW IT IS CANCER.

Later, it is confirmed,

This is the one time as a physician you wish you were wrong.

At times we all get that hunch we cannot explain, it is going to be a certain diagnosis, and then it is that diagnosis and normally you trust that hunch. But this time you wish that hunch was wrong, but it is not.

You have joined the millions of others, you have CANCER.

The six-letter word that I believe now really should have been a four-letter word. The minute you say it, nothing else matters.

It changes your life. Whether contained or not you can never go back.

Survivors are who we are.

We are in an exclusive club that no one wants to join. But once we join, we feel an instant bond with all the other people who have been given that horrible one-word diagnosis. I did not understand this before, but now that I have joined the club, I get it.

Survivors see the world just a little bit differently.

Bad days are not as bad and good days are a little brighter because we understand days can be taken away in an instant.

Mortality has been shown to us, and that has awakened us, allowing us to appreciate the littlest things in life.

We physicians work so hard taking care of our patients,

That sometimes we forget that we may have to look at medicine from the other side of the tracks.

—Laurie Azine

I reply, "Thank you for sharing your poem. That is so meaningful to me!" I wonder if I should tell her I am writing a book about my experiences. I see some of the very same thoughts and phrases appearing in her poem that I have been writing about as of late. *This is the one time as a physician that you wish you were wrong.* I'd love to get her opinion on it; maybe I'll send her an early draft.

If I can resonate with her poem and *Minnesota Monthly* feels it is worthy of publication, perhaps there are others out there who might benefit from my writing, too. Helping patients cope with the nature of an illness, a new diagnosis, potentially confusing or frightening treatment plans—that's what I spent years of my life training to do and continue to do every day.

I just never thought I would accomplish any of it in quite this way.

Chapter 3

You've Got a Friend in Me (Part I): The Women

Cause it's a bittersweet symphony, this life.
—The Verve

I generally do not recommend having to endure a health crisis in order to solidify, extend, or perhaps (on the opposite end) pare down your existing list of friends, mentors, support groups, acquaintances. On the other hand, in the few short months after I was diagnosed with breast cancer, that's exactly what happens.

There is, of course, in the early days, the sheer panic. In the minutes, hours, days after receiving the news, in the wake of the physical and emotional response, who can I turn to? *Help, Lord!* Later, after there is less panic, more actual processing, but still knowing there is a very long journey ahead, who should be in the know, the inner circle? Someone who will actually be supportive and helpful, not just curious or privy to gossip or drama. Who can I count on for the long haul, knowing there is no "right" answer? Here is how it actually played out.

The first few days after I found the breast lump at home, I knew something was amiss. I had a strong sense that whatever came next (scans, biopsies, or more), this was not going to turn out to be something simple or benign. Call it my women's intuition or my physician brain or whatever have you, I had come to the conclusion myself days before the actual mammogram that I had breast cancer. It was a Sunday evening. Sitting up in bed, reading a book, I reach down to scratch an itch on my right chest when I feel this lump underneath my fingertips—soft, smooth, rubbery, but definitely different. The next morning, I would do the same thing in the shower, thinking, *Maybe that was just a bad dream?* But no, it's still there. Monday, midmorning, I call the clinic, and they schedule me for the first available appointment on Tuesday, 8:30 a.m. I tell no one. I am still mulling this over, thinking, *But what if this actually turns out benign? Then I will have put others through unnecessary stress and anxiety, the waiting, the worry.*

The next day, Tuesday, my primary doc is out. Her practice partner is a very nice and rather young family medicine physician who feels the same lump. She frowns, furrows her brow, and orders the mammogram and ultrasound and biopsy that may follow. It's scheduled for Thursday. I leave, go to work for the rest of the day. Again, I tell no one.

Wednesday night is a regularly scheduled evening of activities at my church. There are kids' youth groups, adult Bible studies, choir practice, and so on. Five years ago, I decided to join in. The honest truth? I wanted to drop my young kids off in a program and, yes, I will admit, have someone else take care of them, knowing they will learn about God for an hour and a half while I went upstairs to connect with other women and have real adult conversation, including food, friendship, and fellowship, via the women's Bible study. This may sound selfish, the motivation for it, but it was where I was at and what I needed at the time. Other hipster women get to have their book club. Well, this is *my* book club, the greatest book ever written! Number 1 best seller of all time! Over 5 billion copies sold and distributed!

When I first joined the group of about fifteen to twenty women, I was struck by the diversity of ages—from mid-twenties, newly married, or newly pregnant through upper eighties, facing health issues and decisions about moving into assisted living. I appreciated this very much; one thing I miss about losing both Grandma Helen and Grandma Jeanette in the last five years is not having access to their wisdom and experience and sage advice. Although, sadly, since *both* women were affected by Alzheimer's dementia, the loss came years before their actual death. Still, as I look around the table, I see a wonderful array of kind faces and friendly smiles underneath the gray hair and glasses. There are a few middle-aged ladies, too (single, single again, or married with kids in high school and college), and then there's me, Amanda, and Rachel, the young guns, the newbies, the "girls" as they keep calling us, the three moms of small children. I think to myself, this could be the start of a beautiful group mentoring relationship.

Fast-forward five years, that Wednesday following the clinic appointment but before the actual tests, I am sitting in the very same Bible study, and at the end, we discuss prayer requests. This is the first time I finally open up, and I tell the group I am having a mammogram and possibly a biopsy tomorrow afternoon. I also mention I am fairly certain this is going to be abnormal. They obviously know I am an MD; they seem to take my word for it. Diane, the group leader, immediately responds that she is a breast cancer survivor and asks for a show of hands around the table—six additional women (over 30 percent) raise their hands to say, "Yes, I've had this too." Wow, I am immediately aware of how important this group was to me in the past, and now, going into the future, even more so. Next, I admit to them that I have not even told *my husband* yet; you all are the first to know. Several of them frown; however, these same women are also aware of Paul's struggle with anxiety. We've prayed for this issue. I mention, "I was hoping not to stress him out or add to his anxiety until I knew some actual results were back." I see some heads nodding, a look of sympathy, but still, a slight sense of "Hmmm, not a good idea" hangs in the air. Then a pregnant pause. "Okay, all right," I say, "I will tell him tonight or tomorrow morning, but I am still not taking him to the appointment!" I just didn't relish the idea of him nervously pacing around a waiting room while I am being squashed flat as a pancake in a mammogram machine or enduring the startling cap gun snap of the core biopsy. Heads nod again; Diane offers to go along with me. Later we pray, asking for peace and comfort while waiting on results.

The next morning, I finally do tell Paul that I found a lump in my breast and I am going to have a mammogram today, possibly more if needed. He seems pretty nonchalant about it; he says, "Well, if you think you have found a lump, yes, you should go check it out." I mention that 80 percent of all breast biopsies seller's return policy. Magazines, newspapers, eBooks, digital downloads, and used books are not returnable or exchangeable. Defective NOOKs may be exchanged at the store in accordance with the applicable warranty.

Returns or exchanges will not be permitted (i) after 14 days or without receipt or (ii) for product not carried by Barnes & Noble or Barnes & Noble.com.

Policy on receipt may appear in two sections.

Return Policy

With a sales receipt or Barnes & Noble.com packing slip, a full refund in the original form of payment will be issued from any Barnes & Noble Booksellers store for returns of undamaged NOOKs, new and unread books, and unopened and undamaged music CDs, DVDs, vinyl records, toys/games and audio books made within 14 days of purchase from a Barnes & Noble Booksellers store or Barnes & Noble.com with the below exceptions:

A store credit for the purchase price will be issued (i) for purchases made by check less than 7 days prior to the date of return, (ii) when a gift receipt is presented within 60 days of purchase, (iii) for textbooks, (iv) when the original tender is PayPal, or (v) for products purchased at Barnes & Noble College bookstores that are listed for sale in the Barnes & Noble Booksellers inventory management system.

Opened music CDs, DVDs, vinyl records, audio books may not be returned, and can be exchanged only for the same title and only if defective. NOOKs purchased from other retailers or sellers are returnable only to the retailer or seller from which they are purchased, pursuant to such retailer's or seller's return policy. Magazines, newspapers, eBooks, digital downloads, and used books are not returnable or exchangeable. Defective NOOKs may be exchanged at the store in accordance with the applicable warranty.

Valid through 10/31/2019

Buy 1
Fresh Baked Cookie
Get 1 FREE

Mix or match any flavor.
Try our limited time only
Cookie Monster's Everything Cookie*

To redeem: Present this coupon in the Café.

D4R9D9L

Buy 1 Fresh Baked Cookie Get 1 Free:
Valid for Fresh Baked cookies only.
1 redemption per coupon.
*While supplies last.
Ask Cafe cashier for details.

turn out benign, again trying not to add to his anxiety, but fairly convinced I was going to be in the 20 percent. He seems somewhat reassured. He offers to accompany me, but I tell him, "I have no idea how long this will take or how much they will need to do, and so let's just meet up and discuss afterwards. Maybe grab a coffee or meet at Chianti Grill for dinner if it's later."

While I am at the radiology office at 2:00 p.m. that afternoon by myself near Maplewood Mall, my phone is dinging, getting multiple e-mails and texts from the ladies in my women's Bible study. They are, even in the very moment the biopsy is happening, with me every step of the way. Later on, after the pathology was positive for cancer, I would immediately update the group via e-mail, and of course, every Wednesday evening going forward, I provide more information—the preliminary reports, the oncology appointment, the next steps, and so on. This same group of women sent me a lovely card in the mail in the weeks leading up to surgery, a get-well card with over fifteen handwritten inscriptions inside. I read through their kind words and encouraging sentiments with such gratitude.

After surgery, with lifting and driving restrictions and so on, Amanda offers to pick me up and bring us to church on Wednesdays following the operation. She and other women from Bible study bring meals—a Crock-Pot of roast beef, a chicken-and-rice casserole, a pan of enchiladas. I am almost feeling guilty about all this, all the attention and the support and the extra help, but my Mom reminds me that women need to come together and truly *want* to help out at such a time as this.

Other female friends in my life—some I've had for many years—also become that much more important to me. Jodie, a fellow soprano in the Oratorio Society of Minnesota, a community choir I've been a part of since medical school. Rachel, whom I know through not one but actually three connections: school, Bible study, and a separate moms' group / book club that meets once a month. Monica, whom I met at our former place of worship and the founder of that very same moms' group. And Karin, who was married to Kent, a longtime friend of Paul's, dating all the way back to grade school in Rapid City, South Dakota. They live just blocks away in our neighborhood, and as such, we often bump into each other when out on a bike ride or walking the dog or at the local coffee shop at the end of our block. But suddenly, after the cancer diagnosis, with all these women, our conversations at every turn take on a completely different dynamic and a much deeper meaning.

We talk about things such as fear, anxiety, how to break bad news (or any news at all) to your family, including a husband who might be burying his head in the sand as a coping mechanism. We talk about our children, how they handle adversity, how we role-model coping skills, and how to explain the fact that life is just plain hard even to a nine-year-old whose main concern should be enjoying a warm summer day in the backyard. We discuss physical things like aging, attractiveness, and so on, what it's like adjusting to a completely new self after surgery, and how society and expectations and body image are woven into this fabric no matter how hard one might try to tease it out. We discuss the importance of faith, family, friends, and of course, reaching out to one another in times of need. For us, gone are the days of "So how are you?" followed immediately by "Fine! But just so busy!"

And good riddance to *that*. I'm enjoying, on multiple levels, the much deeper connections, the more meaningful dialogue, the newfound ability to share personal stories, even painful stories, without fear or embarrassment or the sense of self-consciousness one might expect when discussing these sorts of topics. I stop and pause and find myself wondering, *Why did it take a diagnosis of cancer to accomplish all this? Why wait until the fear of death and dying or surgery or chemo or whatever else grips hold of your heart to open up to others?* Maybe, this is God's version of the extreme wake-up call. The shoulder tap. The tugging at the heartstrings reminding us that this is what *really* matters.

> I'll take you down the only road
> I've ever been down . . .
> You know, the one that takes you
> to the places where all things meet,
> yeah...
> —The Verve

Chapter 4

You've Got a Friend in Me (Part II): The Men

This life, this life aches
And this life moans
This life, this life is great
And it's better when you're not alone.
—The Black Crowes

Prior to becoming a mom, I would actually say I had more male friends than female friends throughout college, med school, and into residency. "Why?" one might ask. I am left to ponder. Not sure exactly, but I will venture a guess here, a theory, that at least at a *much earlier* stage in life, without the benefit of age and wisdom and maturity and the common bond of motherhood, women can be harder to get to know than men. Gals at times seem to have a competitive edge, a more complicated emotional terrain, while guys just tend to be more open, honest, tell it like it is. I am not trying to be judgmental, and of course, I am overgeneralizing here quite a bit. I'm simply describing what I observe and what fostered certain relationships for me early on.

One of my best friends in college and medical school—all eight years—was Nick, originally from the small town of Mullen, Nebraska, now a practicing ob-gyn in Littleton, New Hampshire. He and I were great friends, always platonic, and study partners getting through not only the undergraduate biology major and the MCAT but also the preclinical years of medical school, including passing step 1 of the USMLE. While in college, we also carpooled to 3M together, both working as lab techs, different floors, same building. In the first two years of med school, we were even roommates sharing a two-bedroom apartment just south of campus off East River Parkway. Luckily, it also had two full bathrooms, which is the only way this arrangement would have ever worked, given my tendency to monopolize this space for what (others tell me) can seem like hours on end. I guess I can be a bit high maintenance—hair, makeup, and so on. During medical school, we also had two other study buddies, Jeff and Craig. The four of us would review material together as a group, quizzing each other and so on, often over dinner at each other's houses, which made studying much more enjoyable.

Later on, I had another good friend, Bill, as a golf partner, fishing buddy, and sounding board during internal medicine residency. After Paul and I started dating, the three of us would often play nine holes after work since we were all quite fond of the game at the time. This was during the most recent heyday of golf, the peak of Tiger Woods's career, an era when you actually needed a tee time well in advance to play on the weekend. Moving past residency and on to my career as faculty, I kept these male friends and added some new ones in the form of colleagues, getting to know Charlie Moldow and Dave Macomber then Jim Langland quite well as my practice partners. Given they were a bit older than me, they became informal mentors as well—Charlie, of course, in a much deeper and more meaningful way after our recent ordeals. I also made friends with my nurse Tony, going beyond the usual RN/MD working relationship and gaining a closeness and respect for each other's opinions and values that would foster more of true friendship.

After the diagnosis and the stress and strife it introduced, I became acutely aware once again of the importance of friends, both male and female. I think, in particular, the diagnosis of breast cancer carries with it different connotations. So much of what happens next depends on your attitude and worldview and outlook on things such as physical appearance, self-image, self-confidence, sex appeal, and so on, which is inherently different for each and every woman—no one right answer or correct approach but an individualized decision. At the same time, it helps to have advice, input, observations, and support from *both* men and women throughout this endeavor, and not just the spouse or significant other but family and friends as well. There is also somehow a certain sense of validation when your male friends stick up for you, stand by you after enduring this type of a challenge to your femininity, even when it's coming from a completely platonic relationship. I found that I very much needed to seek advice, vent, and unload at times onto the other people in my life, men included. And, I truly appreciated hearing from them that I looked great and that I was still an attractive woman. I needed those reassurances, very much, at that point in time.

Although I must admit, occasionally I thought perhaps it is odd that I *haven't* relied completely on Paul regarding the cancer diagnosis, in terms of the supporting role, the sounding board, and so on. It's complicated, to say the least. Why is it that sometimes I find it easier to talk to Charlie or other people about these issues rather than my own husband? Is this normal?

Well, some of it is Paul's history of anxiety. I was acutely aware of this and truly didn't want to add to his burden of worry by constantly discussing my medical issues, speculating about the future, and so on. Early on, he didn't seem to want to talk about it much around the house. Most questions or concerns I verbalized out loud were met with the suggestion of "Bring it up at your next appointment." The other part of it has to do with Charlie and me being both physicians; we have a high-level baseline medical knowledge. We can move quickly through the details and jump ahead lightning fast to discuss potential implications. Our brains both move forward at the same speed and with similar approaches, similar attitudes toward medical decision-making. Our conversations simply flow naturally, whereas I have to stop and pause and explain so many different aspects to Paul or my mom or my friend Jodie or anyone honestly who hasn't gone through four years of med school, three years of residency, then three years of heme/onc fellowship in Charlie's case. I came to realize how fortunate I am to have these other *physicians* in my life that I can commiserate with in such an easy manner, and not just on a professional level but on a personal level as well.

Speaking of which, it was also quite interesting getting to know Todd Tuttle. At first I thought, is it odd, a bit unusual, to first find out you have cancer, research just about every breast surgeon in the Twin Cities, then come up with the best fit—and it turns out this physician is two floors below you in the same building? Okay, maybe that's *not* really all that unusual. After all, yes, M Health is quite well known for its expertise in cancer care. But then to realize (after meeting a few times and talking with him and discussing issues, and not just my health or my situation but also things such as the university, the new building, academic medicine, hobbies, and outside interests) that the two of us would get along famously, have very similar personalities, similar attitudes toward medicine and academia, and so on, well, *that* was pretty unexpected.

Or was it? I think back to the way I chose him to be my surgeon in the first place. I read through his entire list of publications on PubMed that were anything related to breast cancer. In doing this, I could tell that he had an approach to surgical decision-making that I would value—always evidence-based, rather conservative, don't "do" something just because we can or we think it might have benefit or the patient and family are demanding it. He was also not afraid to take on some of the more controversial issues, such as arguing against contralateral prophylactic mastectomy. And sensing this, I chose him because *I* tend to think this very same way and practice medicine in a similar fashion, and I wanted someone who could think this way *for me* while in the throes of extreme anxiety, having to make decisions at a point in time when I really couldn't reason rationally. In retrospect, it worked out beautifully, exactly what I was hoping for—as in respecting my decision not to reconstruct, gently talking me out of a bilateral mastectomy, having a calm and level-headed approach when I was instead experiencing moments of total panic.

So it should really not be that much of a surprise that, if the two of us think alike in this one particular area, there are going to be other similarities as well. It starts to remind me of how we as physicians really bring our entire persona, our total worldview, into the practice of medicine—such as becoming a mom greatly influenced the way I view certain aspects of patient care. Having a strong faith background makes me think differently about end-of-life issues. And now recently, becoming a patient myself has changed, in very profound ways, how I care for and advocate for my patients as they navigate the same complicated health-care system.

Later on, at some point, I connect with Todd, and we meet at the Campus Club to discuss a paper we are writing together. After almost two hours of talking about everything and nothing, he suddenly says, "Is this weird? That you were once my patient? Do you have patients that you also consider friends?"

To that I reply, "Well, the answer is yes, but just for the record, I am no longer your patient. That's it, I am firing you as my doctor! I have no further need for a surgeon, thank God. But even if I do, you can refer me to your partner, Dr. Jane Hui! That way, we can go back to being colleagues, friends—it'll be much simpler." He just laughs. Perhaps this is not the first time Dr. Todd Tuttle had someone fire him as their doctor, in light of some of his publications and presentations on the controversies surrounding breast cancer management. Thinking more about his question, though, I reach into my purse and produce a small white piece of paper and hand it to him. It's a fortune out of a fortune cookie from our local Chinese restaurant. It reads: "Soon someone new in your life will become a very good friend."

I say, "I think this is you as the only new person in my life, honestly, who could possibly qualify in this way."

He smiles and asks, "Can I keep this?"

I reply, "Yes, of course." He tucks it into his wallet.

And that is the start of yet another cherished male friendship.

Chapter 5

The Book (Chapter) about a Book

> This is my fight song . . .
> Take back my life song . . .
> Prove I'm all right song.
> —Rachel Platten

Writing a book (chapter) about writing a book feels a bit like you are recording a video of someone filming a video—a lens inside a lens inside another lens and so on, ad infinitum. However, in 2016, from first encountering the breast cancer diagnosis on March 31, then starting to write about it on April 17, to sharing early drafts of my manuscript on May 19, to submitting the partial work to publishers in mid-June, and finally finishing my first book at midnight on August 6, well, this has been such a transforming force in my life. It simply cannot be ignored or left out of the story.

Early on, the book was meant to simply capture the memories, a memoir of sorts, writing everything down—the good, the bad, the ugly, the positive, including some of the amazing connections and "coincidences." This would help me remember everything before I might forget some of the details. Later, it became very therapeutic, a way for me to get the thoughts and ideas and emotions out of my head and onto paper and, therefore, stop having to play them over in my mind time and again. Another benefit: at times when I would question some of my decisions, it was helpful to go back and read those early chapters and remind myself why. Or later, when contemplating the possibility of a follow-up MRI, I would go back and reread "The MRI Saga" to remember some of the ridiculousness that goes along with this entire process, and laugh.

Somewhere near end of May or early June, the book took on an entirely different dynamic. I noticed that I started to write less about me and more about my patients, my students, my training as a doctor. It started to coalesce into a story, as opposed to a journal. It became a force unto itself. Then, in different stages, phases, ever-widening concentric circles if you will, I started to let people read it. First, it was those who were already "in" on the story, close to it, part of my medical world, then later family, then soon after friends, then acquaintances outside the medical world, and so on. Why?

First and foremost, I wanted to get opinions, feedback, and critique from these beta testers. I honestly didn't know—was this going to be something beneficial or perhaps mildly entertaining for others to read, or is this just dear-diary, tell-all, let-it-all-hang-out, chick-lit type drivel? Should it simply stay on my Google Drive for all time as tangible evidence of my own coping skills, or could it possibly be something more?

Also, early on, the rather surprising part for me was to learn about and observe other people's reactions to it. I first gave a paper copy to Paul; he's not very tech-driven; he refuses to own a smartphone, so sending it via a Google link or shared Google doc would probably be met with some degree of obfuscation. I printed it out, the first eighteen chapters, two-sided, put it in a black three-ring binder, and gave it to him right before I left town for Baltimore to present at an academic meeting. I thought, *Perfect timing! I'll be gone for four days. He'll be stuck at the house the entire time, watching the kids. This will give him something to do, and he can read it in my absence and get a better sense of what I've been going through the past few weeks.* Upon my return, we are sitting out on the back patio with Sam and Lydia. I am telling them about my trip and showing them pictures on my phone when suddenly I remember and I say to Paul excitedly, "Hey! What did you think of my book? Please tell me, I'm dying to know!"

He says, "Oh, *that*, well, I haven't even looked at it yet."

Boom. I think I could have reached into my chest, torn out my heart, and tossed it on the bluestone patio beneath our feet. My gaze locks on him. I set down my glass of iced tea, stare back intently, and demand, "Why not?"

"Oh, come on, this is something just for you," he says. "To be writing this down, a dear-diary sort of thing, it's too personal. It should really be for your eyes only."

Okay, but that's the entire point. I wanted you to read it to see if others might benefit from it.

"And besides," he says, "I've been hearing all these stories from you anyway. I don't need to read again about the biopsy and the MRI and surgery and whatnot."

Well, not really. You may think you know the full story, but there is much, much more in this book than what I have been regaling you with the past month.

And lastly, he says, "It's too depressing. I don't want to spend my days reading about cancer."

Whoa, you've got it all wrong. There's a lot of humor in it. That's the part I really enjoy the most.

I'm still reeling in the shock and awe and disappointment that he doesn't want to read something that means this much to me, that is slowly becoming my pet project, my "baby," and has consumed so much of my time, late nights and early mornings. Once, Lydia said goodnight to me as I was typing away at my kitchen table on a Friday evening. Later that night, I turned in around 11:00 p.m. The next morning, after my usual 5:00 a.m. wake-up time, I went downstairs, poured a cup of coffee and went back to the very same spot and started writing again. She emerged from her bedroom at 8:00 a.m. and came into the kitchen with sleepy eyes and wild hair. She yawned then looked at me. Her mouth dropped, and she exclaimed, "Mom! Have you been up all night?" I laughed, thinking well, no, but pretty darn close. I told her, "I'm pulling all-nighters again, just like in college." Having insomnia—early on from the stress and anxiety and later from a tamoxifen-induced menopause—this has helped me accomplish quite a bit of writing, to be sure. A silver lining. Lemonade out of lemons.

Back to the story of the *story.* Later, I calm down, realizing I probably overreacted a bit to Paul's reluctance to read it. He is really not one to read much in the way of fiction or creative memoir for that matter; he prefers books on architecture, philosophy, and theology. And honestly, I have heard similar comments since from other breast cancer survivors: I might *not* want to read this and have to relive the experience all over again. He may come around and read it later, I reasoned, after the dust has settled. But the very next morning, the first day back after Baltimore is also the same day as Charlie's surgery. I am getting ready to leave for work when I pass by the black three-ring binder sitting forlornly on the dining-room table, as if it were feeling slighted, ignored. Suddenly I think, *Aha! Charlie!* He's essentially a captive audience. He'll be stuck in the hospital, recovering from an operation. What better way to pass the time than to be the very first person to read my book? And knowing he is an avid reader himself, belonging to a book club and so on, he might actually crack open the front cover and take a peek at it. Besides, I've written about him extensively in this thing. I will need to know if he is okay with all this, using his name and sharing stories about work and family and even health issues and so on.

Later that same day at the hospital, I will stop by 3C and spend some time with Gay in the patient family waiting area while Charlie's still in the PACU, waiting for a bed on 7C. Gay and I spend well over an hour talking, catching up, and discussing both Charlie's situation and our own health issues in addition to life and coping and the family dynamic. Elaine, the RN assigned to Charlie's recovery, comes out into the waiting area to give us an update. "He's doing great. He is already up and walking around. We are just waiting for a bed on 7C." Then she turns to Gay and says, "Charlie's been asking for his book."

Gay nods, bends over, and starts rummaging around in her tote bag when I interrupt this process, saying, "Wait, no, he's really looking for *this*." And out of my sack, I produce the mysterious black three-ring binder and hand it to her. Both Elaine and Gay glance at it, then turn to look at me quizzically. I say, "Never mind, just give it to him. I'll explain later."

I'm heading out, and on the drive home, I need to stop and pick up dinner. I'm getting home much later than is typical for me. After finishing up and putting away the dishes, I open my tablet

and check e-mail, and there is a very short and cryptic message
from Gay, sent at 8:08 p.m. on that May 19:

> Charlie says, "This is REALLY GOOD,"
> wants to send to his sister the
> publisher, loves the fact that he's in
> it, has some suggestions.

I almost break down in tears, I am so happy. Validation!
Someone actually reads my book and likes it! It turns out he's
read the entire thing, cover to cover, while still in the PACU.
He later tells me he laughed out loud several times; he didn't
know I had such a wicked sense of humor. He does send it right
away to his sister, who, I had almost forgotten, is a publisher at
Simon and Schuster. She has a senior editor review it, Michelle,
who sends me a detailed critique, including areas to improve
and develop further, suggestions for revising or annotating the
medical terminology, potential target audiences. Overall, she
seems impressed, saying, "It's not your usual cancer memoir," but
then politely declines taking it on—not surprising for a first time,
unagented author with a partial manuscript in hand. Instead,
she sends me two more names, other literary agents, but also
mentions that the book has so much local color, I really should be
looking around in the Twin Cities for a local publisher.

So in that very short span of time, I have gone from seriously
contemplating hitting the Delete button to cold calling agents in
the New York City publishing world and sending them a link to
my Google doc. One very interesting thing about Google Docs is
that you can see from your Google Drive when someone else is in
it, reading it. If they are not linked to your Google account, they
will show up as an anonymous icon with the name of an animal
attached to it. I laugh when I am furiously typing away and
suddenly I see Anonymous Fox appear at the top of the document.
Or later Anonymous Skunk, Anonymous Bear. I notice they are
all woodland animals. I ponder, *What does this mean exactly? Is
there a hidden message? Am I missing the forest for the trees?* Nah, I
decide, it's just Google's way of messing with me.

This very helpful boost of confidence from Charlie, it has
quite an effect on me. I decide to start sharing the book with other

people. My RN, Tony, who I think would appreciate some of the references to the importance of having nurses on the team. Todd Tuttle, as my surgeon, featured prominently in the first half. Early on, I get the sense that he might appreciate some of the humor in it; he strikes me as the type of guy who can laugh at himself or laugh at a situation that could seem rather bleak and depressing. It turns out I am completely correct on that one. At the same time my mom reads it, and of course, she loves it. What mother wouldn't feel that way? But I am cautiously optimistic; I appreciate the fact that she's also a member of a book club and very well read herself. Next, I start to let some of my nonmedical friends read it—Jodie first, then Karin, then Amanda. After all, I'm concerned that it might be too medically focused, too technical for the average reader to fully benefit from the story. They do mention occasional difficulty with the jargon but report they still very much enjoy the read.

The most positive aspect of all for me, though, the truly amazing part of it, was then watching how the book served to transform, to deepen, to strengthen even further my relationship with the person reading it, the bond of friendship that was there or was just starting to begin with. In fact, I reason, even if the thing *never* gets published, that's worth it right there. I hear comments such as "I feel as though I know you so much better now," "Wow, I had no idea you grew up in rural Minnesota," "I really enjoyed reading about your kids and how they handled the news," or "My favorite part was how this changed your interactions with patients." Even the sensitive areas that I wrote about, thinking maybe they were just TMI—no, not at all. In fact, it seems the openness and honesty brought many people, especially the women in my life, even closer. We now just have that much more to talk about over coffee or out on our walk. Tony, in clinic, starts sharing private jokes with me about hot flashes or the fact that I briefly wanted to get a tattoo; we have a good laugh even if nobody else understands what we are talking about. My friendship with Karin also deepened significantly. Prior to this, I considered her merely an acquaintance, more a part of my husband's circle; now, I consider her one of my best friends. We go on weekend bike rides together, attend women's Bible study every Wednesday, and plan girls' night out every now and then to go hear live music.

I even venture a guess that perhaps reading my book was how the friendship began between Todd Tuttle and me. Early on, one afternoon, the two of us were sitting at the Beacon near campus, having lunch; we met specifically to discuss the book. I wanted to get his feedback on it, as well as ask permission for me to share personal observations about him, even using his full name for something all the world could read. I had been wracking my brain over the past several weeks, trying to come up with pseudonyms for the entire cast of characters, the multiple physicians I mention in so many different contexts such as Todd, Charlie, Anne Blaes; but I was truly drawing a blank. Then he says, "Go ahead, you can use my name. I'm fine with it." And at that point, I have a memory, a flashback, something embroiled on my brain: me entering his name into the search function in PubMed, then later Google, and reading everything he's published to get a better sense of him as a surgeon.

I say, "Well, as you know, Todd, prior to meeting you in clinic, I had read everything you ever wrote about breast cancer. Now, ironically, as it turns out, you've just read everything *I've* ever written about breast cancer."

He laughs. I'm getting a much better sense of him as a person now, too—and likely vice versa. Another testimony to the power of the written word.

> And I don't really care, if nobody else believes . . .
> 'Cause I've still got a lot of fire left in me.
> —Rachel Platten

Chapter 6

MAROONED (PART I)

Great hospitals do two things. They look after patients,
and they teach young doctors.
—David Ogilvy

D espite the generalized fear and trepidation about
inpatient rounding, I find that I was really looking
forward to one week of attending end of June, my very
first one after medical leave. This is likely because I only attend
a few weeks a year at this point; I keep trying to back out of
inpatient medicine, thinking outpatient clinic is so much more
manageable and predictable, and that's really what I need in
my life right now with two kids and their crazy schedules and
whatnot. But then, after some time, I start to miss hospital work.
The grass is always greener, I guess, but also, I find the complexity
and acuity challenging in a good way. I feel like a "real doctor" on
the wards, honestly, as opposed to evaluating yet another patient
with a viral cold in clinic. So what I have been doing as of late
is backfilling the inpatient schedule when they desperately need
someone because they have a couple of hospitalists leave and the
new hires don't start until two months later, or there is a week
assigned to someone who later decides they are going to travel
for an international rotation, or they secure a grant and are now
devoting all their time to research. This sort of thing is happening
constantly in the academic world. As a result, I get to "dabble"
in hospital medicine, rounding six to eight weeks per year as
opposed to a full-time hospitalist. And this seems to be just the

right amount to keep up those inpatient skills; it is a bit like riding a bike. Once you get it down, it never leaves you. And I feel the two skill sets are very complementary to each other; rounding in the hospital makes me a better clinic doc and vice versa.

The inpatient teams years ago were organized into Maroon (teaching services) and Gold (nonteaching services) after the University of Minnesota colors. The hiring of hospitalists led to a rapid expansion of the inpatient census, and we had to add teams—first Maroon 1–4, then Gold 1 and Gold 2, and now there is even a Gold 3, and you guessed it, Maroon 5. There have been numerous references to Adam Levine since the creation of this additional team staffed with one senior resident and one hospitalist. The residents have also started to refer to being on service as "Marooned." It is a bit legendary, in a sense, as a more challenging inpatient block, compared to the other two hospital sites of the VA and Regions.

Our patients tend to mimic what most community physicians would be managing in the ICU. We have a large liver transplant population; patients with end-stage liver disease are a house of cards. They are fine one minute, then the next, near comatose from hepatic encephalopathy or hypotensive from candida sepsis or, the real scary stuff, upper GI bleeding. The single most terrifying code I ever attended as faculty was my patient who had both end-stage liver and end-stage kidney disease, and when they called a code blue to dialysis, I just knew it was him. I had a sixth sense about it when I had rounded about an hour earlier. He was also being treated for fungal pneumonia. I run down to dialysis, second floor of Mayo, and the patient is simply exsanguinating. First hemoptysis, presumably from the pulmonary nodules, followed by copious amounts of hematemesis—an esophageal variceal bleed, no doubt. I have never seen so much blood in a hospital bed or any hospital room for that matter in my life; it was like something out of a horror movie. I started calling for a Minnesota tube, the last-ditch effort to tamponade the flow invented right here at our home institution. But soon we lost a pulse. The intern, Tyler, began chest compressions, cracking three ribs, which sliced through his glove and right into his hand, exposing him to hepatitis C and immediately buying him several months' worth of follow up appointments for labs and potentially medication. Definitely not one of my favorite moments to recall from my inpatient experiences, but it is embroiled on my brain nonetheless. And it makes me appreciate how serious and rapid gastrointestinal bleeding can be.

Back to the here and now. I am scanning my calendar and looking ahead to the third week in June which is when I start rounding with my inpatient medicine team. The night before, I get a call from the hospitalist, signing out the service of 10 patients and reviewing the plan of care for a seamless transition. The very first morning, I head over from my office in the Mayo Building to meet the team on Unit 5A, and the route that I usually take is the skyway from the fourth floor of Mayo. This skyway then magically becomes the third floor of the hospital moving right past the familiar 3C perioperative area, the operating rooms, the patient family waiting room. Even as I wait to get on the elevator, the doors are opening to the right of me with a full view into the main surgical area, including the electronic OR schedule. So now for this entire week, each and every morning, as I am walking over to start attending rounds at 8:30 a.m., of course, I am having flashbacks to the entire scenario on April 26. I envision sitting in the lounge with Paul, watching early morning CNN, waiting to be called back. Later I remember being wheeled back high on midazolam through those corridors, scanning the floral prints on the walls. Or, I recall waking up groggy in the PACU, trying to force my eyes open as I heard voices coming from the surgical team. I even think back to Charlie and his operation and sitting with Gay in that third-floor lounge for almost two hours, talking about life and health and death and everything in between. Early in the week, I will round on two patients on 7C, and as I pass the room where Charlie stayed overnight, I think back to those times and recall once again the whirlwind of happenings, coincidences, connections. Later in the week, I will need to check on a patient of ours in the PACU who is waking up from anesthesia for a TIPS procedure. I will find her wearing that Bair Hugger, and I see the same RN, Elaine, who took care of me until 3:00 p.m. that afternoon. It's pretty intense, honestly, this feeling of déjà vu, almost distracting. But now, for the very first time since surgery, I must be present in the hospital again (both mentally and physically) for an entirely different reason—to teach, lead a team, and help manage the complex patients. I must simply shake my head and rid my brain of these silvery, ethereal strands of cobwebs in order to focus on more important matters at hand.

I first meet Justin (he's at the very tail end of his first year of residency) and Brendan, the brand-new third-year medical student. Talk about different ends of the spectrum. Justin's great, very skilled and competent managing patients, as one should be by the end of the intern year. But I can tell, he's just a little tired, a little burned out. I sense, on day 1, since we are not admitting new patients that his primary goal is to get out of the hospital as soon as possible. I can't blame him. At this point in my career, I am rounding maybe six weeks total in twelve months, and he's been in the hospital for fully half the calendar year or twenty-six weeks, four weeks at a time, alternating with ambulatory blocks. However, as I think about him and observe his fatigue, I don't even mention the fact that when I was an intern I was assigned ten months of inpatient, one month of ER, and one month of ambulatory care. Those ten months, overnight call every fourth night, working every single weekend, no duty-hour restrictions; sometimes I cannot believe I survived it. But I am trying not to become one of those resentful "back in *my* day" types of attendings. Yes, I learned a lot in a very short period, but as a physician, I am still very much acquiring new knowledge and skills daily to this day, and I am now getting eight hours of sleep a night—well, more like six since going through medical menopause, but still. We don't need to run people into the ground to become competent physicians. We can all learn from our mistakes, even the profession as a whole.

Instead, I respond to Justin a bit differently. There are medicine attendings who will round all morning and into the afternoon and make for a really long day—not me. Life is too short for that, and believe me—given my recent experiences, I feel even more strongly about this than ever before. I tell him, "We are done rounding by 11:00 a.m. come hell or high water, and I will see any remaining patients on my own." He immediately brightens up on that suggestion. The third-year student Brendan is not burned out yet (thank God!). Instead, he's the opposite, all wide-eyed and enthusiastic and interested and engaged. And I think, I can harness that potential too. When we see that one of our liver-failure patients needs a paracentesis that day, Justin sighs and says, "Well, can we meet up after rounds to do this?"

I say, "Brendan's our man. He's going to do it. I will supervise, and I will throw in the procedure note while you are freed up to finish notes and orders on the other patients."

Now, with that in mind, Justin's in a really good mood, and Brendan as well—after all, he gets to take a crack at his very first bedside paracentesis! I skipped the "see one" and went right to "do one" (then teach one)—although he did watch an online video, so I guess that counts. I tell him, "I'm old school. I trained before ultrasound, but luckily, Justin here completed our bedside ultrasound course and can mark the pocket of ascites fluid for us." The two of us successfully drained eight liters at the bedside, and the patient did great, feeling a huge relief of abdominal distension and shortness of breath afterward. The next morning, on rounds, the new senior resident Caroline also joins us. Brendan shares that all the third-year students on the other Maroon teams are jealous of him and his opportunity to do a procedure—that truly makes my day.

The other big time-saver for us on rounds is my tablet because when we are all standing outside the patient's room in the hallway, debriefing on the overnight events or discussing care plans as a team, I can view on my tablet or even on my phone the Epic application known as Canto for Apple or Haiku for Android. I was one of several physicians who signed up to pilot this program over six months ago. It's a way to view information in Epic without having to navigate the entire EMR on a tablet device in a web browser. I tried that before and quickly gave up because it's such a big and multifaceted program—it just doesn't work. With the app, it teases out only the most useful clinical information in a simplified format. Customizable, too, as to what you want to view, whether it's your clinic schedule or the list of patients currently in the ER or a team list, such as Maroon 2.

So this is perfect for rounds. We don't necessarily need to enter orders; we just need to quickly view the vital signs, the med list, and the morning labs. I can even send staff messages through this app. My resident will say, "We really should notify the primary doc that the patient was admitted." I open a staff message, type a quick note, and tell the team, "Yep, it's done already." We marvel at the ease of getting tasks accomplished. Our team rounds were faster than any other medicine service, and this is a big reason why. Now I start to wonder why this feels so very different from using a tablet device in clinic for a patient check-in process. I pause, and I contemplate if there is something we can learn from this endeavor to apply to outpatient medicine.

And I am once again reminded of the need to use technology to improve patient care. At the very least, I am helping the team get things done, improve efficiency, and yes, assist them in getting out of the hospital to enjoy a nice warm summer day in mid-June. And for me, it's not just about expediting rounds. If I can preserve a bit of their sanity and prevent burnout, if I can somehow make things better for a tired and worn-out intern such as Justin, this could have much more meaning in the long run.

As it turns out, burnout in physicians is something quite real and significant. And not just during residency. The impact of long hours, stressful work environments, lack of autonomy, difficult decision-making, and bad patient outcomes (whether there was a medical error or not)—they can all take their toll, year after year, over a thirty- or forty-year career. Burnout manifests in many ways, from cutting back or being unable to practice, to even taking one's own life. The suicide rate for physicians has been estimated as 40 per 100,000. In the overall population, it is 12 per 100,000. This means that physicians are three times as likely to kill themselves as the general population, yet this issue is not very widely discussed. Compare: the suicide rate for veterans is around 30 per 100,000. This seems to garner much more publicity. Each issue is equally important, of course, but until we start to pay attention as a profession and start to care for the caretakers themselves, I wonder how we'll ever move forward. And this honestly starts to feel like an extension of my entire worldview after being diagnosed with cancer. Let's focus on what is important, what is essential, what is high yield. Let's keep what we, as doctors, love about medicine, and let's try to minimize the stuff we don't.

My husband, not being part of the medical world, keeps saying that if I were in private practice and not academic medicine, I'd make more money and have more control over my time. Money, perhaps. Control? Definitely not, at least not in this current marketplace and practice environment. Because at the University of Minnesota, our academic physicians—*at least for now*—are not held to a strict productivity model, in part because we wear so many hats. I personally feel I have a lot of autonomy and control over my schedule; I can decide (within reason, of course) how much time I want to devote to teaching versus administrative roles versus patient care. And that, more than anything else, has greatly improved my job satisfaction, as well as my mental health. It's my number one biggest fear with the discussions around health system mergers, regarding the future, that as a part of some deal we will all be forced to conform to one practice model, one way of doing things. The focus would be on finances or productivity, not accounting for situations such as having a medical student or resident with you in clinic, or running a research lab, or needing to submit a grant by a certain deadline. We have heard that the new organizational leadership, including the board of directors and CEO and such, will be a partnership of *academic physicians*. I sincerely hope that this is the case, and that small issues with big implications—such as a lack of autonomy leading to physician burnout—are not lost in transition.

However, rather than facing burnout, our team seems to be getting along very well and really enjoying themselves, even on just day 2. Justin has a sharp wit and a cynical sense of humor, and I very much appreciate that. We joke around quite often on rounds. Three of our patients have some sort of wound management going on, post-surgical, and when he asks me my opinion, I inform him I don't do wounds, thinking, *I've had enough of that over the past two months, thank you.* I also tell him the old doctor joke: "How do you hide a hundred-dollar bill from an internist? Place it under a dressing." He laughs and responds, "We'll call surgery, or have the wound nurses come by." Caroline, the senior resident, is medicine-pediatrics, which actually comes in very handy when we admit an adult with congenital adrenal hyperplasia; she's extremely bright. I can tell it's going to be a good week.

On Tuesday, also trying to boost their morale, I take them all to lunch at the Campus Club at Coffman Union when noon conference is canceled. We all get to enjoy some good food and great conversation. We talk about career plans. Justin says, "I'm considering GI versus hospitalist medicine." I respond, "Well, you are certainly in the right place. Both are very strong in our residency program!" Brendan is trying to decide between internal medicine and emergency medicine. I give him the name of a faculty member at Hennepin County Medical Center. Dr. Richard Gray, who trained in a combined IM/EM program, is a great teacher and diagnostician himself and would make a great mentor. Since I was a student, he's risen to program director. I emphasize to them the importance of mentorship, thinking back to how much it has meant to me over the years and definitely even more over the past few months. *If only they knew how much.*

But eventually, these young doctors will discover it for themselves, just as I did; I only hope sooner rather than later and ideally under much more pleasant circumstances. Interestingly, mentorship has also been found in a number of studies to have a protective effect against burnout. Makes sense, and that's another strategy right there to ensure that residents and also early career faculty—two of the more difficult periods in our training—are well connected with mentors.

I go back to my office, later in the day, to co-sign notes in the EMR and submit the billing. I look through my desk drawer, this time past the thank-you notes and other blank cards and into an area where I keep my business cards. One is for my patients; it lists the contact numbers to the clinic, the phone and fax, as well as the days I am in clinic. Another is more of an academic business card—listing my name, my title, my email address, office phone number, and pager. I decide to take one academic card with me and give it to Brendan at the end of the week. Maybe he'll change his mind and decide he wants to pursue internal medicine; I've swayed a few students over the years. It's another opportunity I don't want to miss if it leads to something more significant down the road.

Chapter 7

Marooned (Part II)

Getting out of the hospital is a lot like resigning
from a book club. You're not out of it
until the computer says you're out of it.
—Erma Bombeck

On Wednesday, we are on "long call," which means admitting patients until 6:00 p.m. We have a few admissions over the course of the day—a new admit from the ER with pneumonia, a transfer from an outside hospital with complicated pancreatitis. Later in the afternoon, I get a call from the triage doc about an admission from clinic. He's also an MD, a staff cardiologist at a local hospital with some very abnormal labs; he's got rising bilirubin after finishing a course of antibiotics for pneumonia after traveling to Morocco. Wow, what a differential diagnosis we have going here, a very long list of potential etiologies. And are the two related or two separate distinct entities? I am also hearing symptoms from the clinic doc that I really don't like, such as fevers and unexplained weight loss. My inner red flags are going up. We need to discuss the case with multiple consult teams, including gastroenterology, infectious disease.

But later, when I am back in the team room with the intern, resident, and student, what comes up in this particular discussion is trying to care for a physician as a patient. I sit back and listen to the astute observations coming from them. Justin says, "I am really worried that this guy has cancer. He seems to minimize his symptoms, typical MD. He took so long to come in for evaluation—colleagues were telling him he was jaundiced, for God's sake!" I think, *Denial, perhaps? Knowing too much? Physician brain working against you? Not wanting to get the scan for fear of what it might actually show?* They also contemplate, "Could he be more of a drinker than he lets on?" Again, thinking about physician stress and burnout, inwardly I reflect, *I am glad they are least considering this possibility.*

Of course, ID and GI both see him right away. They recommend ordering a slew of labs, viral hepatitis serologies, along with some autoimmune antibodies and inflammatory markers. Unfortunately, most of these labs will take several days to return. They also want to proceed with an MRI of the pancreas and liver. This is scheduled for first thing the next morning.

Midafternoon of the next day, I decide to stop by his room just by myself and have a talk with this attending cardiologist. I sit down next to the bedside; his daughter Marie is with him. She's not medically trained but says, "I learn by osmosis." I relay to both of them the tentative plans: "Even though your bilirubin is still rising, we could discharge you home because you have no new symptoms, and the MRI was fairly unremarkable." The subspecialists are attributing this all to drug-induced cholestasis. Apparently, it happens with Augmentin, which is the antibiotic he was prescribed to treat pneumonia. "We see this" is what they keep saying. There are several case reports in the literature as well; the team is very reluctant to perform a biopsy or anything more invasive. It will take time; the jaundice will slowly resolve. Which is fine, it very well may be the case, but as a general internist and not a subspecialist, my mind always goes to plan B. What if the bilirubin continues to rise? What if new, additional LFT abnormalities develop? What about the weight loss and fevers? Were they related to pneumonia or something more insidious?

So while in the room with the patient and his daughter, I decide to ask him a new and different line of questioning; "What is your worst fear regarding this illness?" He pauses, stares out the window at the Mississippi River, avoiding my gaze, then says, "Well, I don't think I have a malignancy based on my scans, but my wife died of pancreatic cancer five years ago." He goes to say she was a patient here at the university, diagnosed with stage 4 initially, and only lived for another month after that. I ponder the meaning of this fact. "Painless jaundice," which is exactly what my cardiologist has right now, is a hallmark presentation of pancreatic cancer. How awful he must have felt, turning yellow from head to toe with that working medical knowledge and harrowing personal experience in his mind. No wonder he put off coming in to be evaluated. I can understand a bit better what might be going through his head.

Then he turns to look at me and says, "What are *you* most worried about at this point?" Wow, what a conversation we are having. I hesitate at first. Do I tell him I'm still concerned about other potential etiologies, or will that undermine his confidence in the GI team's assessment? Do I just say, "Yes, I agree with our experts, we're sending you home," and be done with it? Then suddenly I think back to Gay Moldow and one of her email messages. She says: "Tell us what to expect, whether it's going to be good or bad. The caregiver and patient need information. We don't care good or bad, we just need to know!!!!!"

So I take a deep breath, and I say: "Imaging is just imaging. Sometimes we rely too much on one scan or one particular test." While it is true that his MRCP was "unremarkable," it was not perfectly normal either; there are several focal pancreatic cysts, a few slight abnormalities that may need follow-up. So next I say, "I have to admit I am still a bit concerned about malignancy, potentially pancreatic, but also cholangiocarcinoma. It could also be a new presentation of primary biliary cirrhosis/cholangitis." All these entities would require a tissue diagnosis; he would need either a liver biopsy or an ERCP scope with endoscopic brush biopsies. He slowly nods, looks over toward his daughter, then back at me. I am pretty sure I am the only physician on multiple teams to have mentioned the *c-word* to him. Is this just because I have cancer on the brain lately? I sincerely hope it is not clouding my clinical judgment. However, if it were me, I would want to know that these thoughts were running through the mind of the attending physician in charge of my care. I emphasize that these potential diagnoses are much less likely but might be considered on follow-up.

He says, "Well, I came here to get the expertise of the U, especially the opinion from GI. You are a liver transplant center, after all, and I know you see unusual cases all the time."

I tell him, "Yes, you are in very good hands." I mention I will send a staff message to Dr. Jack Lake, the hepatologist with the most clinical experience regarding liver disease of any type. I've sent him staff messages before and he always replies promptly. It will be an easy way to get a second opinion while we are waiting for more labs to come back. And then I decide to go out on a limb: "I've had my own health issues recently, too, and came here to the U, seeking care from my own colleagues. It was a bit awkward at first, but I got over it, simply because I wanted the very best team."

They both nod and express their appreciation, both for his care and the care his wife received here so many years ago. He asks me, "Have you ever practiced anywhere else?"

I say, "No, the U really has their hooks in me now. A loyal Golden Gopher to the day I die, I guess."

But back to the discharge plan. If I can't perform a liver biopsy myself or be the physician who does the ECRP, then I revert back to what I do best: schedule close follow-up in clinic. I whip out my mobile phone and right in the room, at 2:55, I send a text to my nurse, Tony. "Hey there! I need you to schedule an appointment with me next Tuesday, a Mr. Daniels, MR number 0051687433, hospital follow-up." At 2:56, he texts back: "Done! 4:00 p.m." I ask the patient and his daughter if this date and time works, and they immediately reply, "We'll be there," and proceed to both thank me repeatedly, about six times each, while vigorously shaking my hand.

So at least following up and with tincture of time, we will know. If he has a malignancy or an autoimmune disorder or something that is just not yet apparent on imaging, eventually, he will present with more symptoms or worsening labs, *something* to alert us that this is not just Augmentin. And if it's just an unfortunate side effect of the medication, then it will also be self-evident and simply improve over time.

I go back to the team room and fill in the residents about the new plan to discharge him today, and guess what—I've already secured an appointment with me in clinic next week! I'm remembering the importance of actually *having* a date and time, as it certainly was for me and later for Charlie, and not just "follow up with primary care in one to two weeks." I show them the text on my phone from Tony. There are two other hospitalists sitting in the team room—the triage doc and also the attending on Maroon 1. Neither of them has seen a patient in the ambulatory setting since residency. They are overhearing me tell the entire story, and I say to Justin, "Now, aren't you glad that your attending is a traditional internist who also has outpatient clinic? I don't think any hospitalist can expedite a discharge quite like that!" We all share in a laugh. The triage doc is staring at the computer in front of him but looks over at me with a smirk on his face and rolls his eyes.

I'm feeling very good about the series of events that just occurred, and I cannot help but wonder if it would have turned out the same way without my recent experiences to guide me. For a moment in time, I am actually grateful I had the opportunity to become a patient. I want to let it change me, influence my practice style, mold me and shape me, stretch me and grow me. Because if my ten-year survival rate is really 95 percent, then that's a lot of time left potentially to continue to experience the transforming effects. Perhaps many patients under my care—and even these young doctors in training—could really benefit from this, God-willing. Maybe that's worth it in the end.

Chapter 8

Marooned (Part III)

Cure sometimes, treat often, comfort always.
—Hippocrates

The week of inpatient attending is flying by. The pace of hospital medicine is definitely a fast-moving one. We round in the morning, often do procedures late morning or early afternoon, then tuck in the ICU transfers and holdovers and later, new admissions then suddenly you look up at the clock and it's after 6:00 p.m. Where did the time go? It's a whirlwind, a blur, enjoyable but all-consuming and a bit tiring. There's a reason we only attend for one or two weeks at a time in the hospital.

On Friday morning, we are back on long call again, and early on we take two holdovers admitted by the night float the night before. We are heading over to 5A, and we stop outside the patient's room. I have not heard one word yet about either admission; I have only seen their names pop up on my team list in Epic. So far, we have nine patients; the team cap is twelve, so we will admit three more later in the day. Our census includes three patients with end-stage liver disease, two patients with pancreatitis, a lung-transplant patient with worsening renal function, a woman with COPD and pneumonia, and a heroin abuser with right-sided endocarditis. Justin the intern has taken over from night float, and he begins presenting the new patient.

"This is a fifty-year-old female whose only past medical history is breast cancer. She had, I believe, a right mastectomy with lymph node removal within the past year. This has been complicated by arm swelling, lymphedema of the right arm; and last night, she came in with increasing arm pain, redness, and a fever. Her blood cultures are already positive for group B strep. There appears to be a small cut on her right hand, which may have been the portal of entry for a cellulitis."

He stops and looks at me. I am wondering about the expression on my face; I literally had to lean up against the wall upon hearing this. First, let me explain. In over fifteen years of attending, I have not admitted a patient with a breast-cancer-related complication; they are typically managed by our inpatient oncology service. Even my own clinic patients who have breast cancer and are hospitalized for infection or anemia or a host of other concerns—they are on 7D, not on the general medicine service. So first I think, *Why is she on Maroon?* And second I think, *Good Lord, what are the chances that a patient with breast cancer would be admitted by night float and then transferred to <u>my team</u> out of the seven possible admitting medicine services? More irony, more strange coincidences. What on earth is going on? Bizarre things just keep happening to me. And indeed, it's the right arm, is it? Huh, just like me. Is this a harbinger of things to come? Cellulitis, group B strep bacteremia from just a tiny cut . . . the physical therapist warned me to protect my arm.* These thoughts are simply racing around in my head as I stand there, saying nothing.

Next, I realize that my entire team is looking at me—the intern, the resident, the medical student, the pharmacy student. They are waiting for me to say something. I am really, quite honestly, having a moment here. I stare back, I don't know whether to laugh, cry, walk away; so I just stand there, shaking my head. Obviously, they don't know. I haven't said anything; they can't possibly realize that I am only eight weeks out from a right mastectomy myself and now recently having problems with my right arm. The irony of the situation is totally lost on them. But I have got to snap out of it. I am still standing there, dumbstruck, for probably thirty seconds or more. I've got to think of some logical response.

I say, "Well, Group B strep is a bit of a strange organism."
That is true. It's not the first bug I associate with cellulitis or
soft tissue infections, but later, doing a lit search, we will find
out lymphedema is a risk factor. Justin replies, "We've got her
on cefazolin and gent." I say, "Did she have an axillary lymph
node dissection or sentinel lymph node biopsy?" He's not sure. I
tell him "That's okay; we will review the chart or simply ask the
patient." I recognize it's hard picking up holdovers from night
float. You just don't quite have all the details in your head as if you
admitted the patient yourself. He lists off her home medications.
At first, he states, "Tamoxifen," and then says, "Oh wait, no, she
was switched to the other one."

I say, "An aromatase inhibitor."

He replies, "Yes, that's it. Letrozole."

As far as the arm is concerned, I tell him, "We should probably
consult our lymphedema therapists and have them come by right
away. It's Friday, after all, not sure they round on either Saturday
or Sunday."

I am still completely dazed and confused, but finally, I snap
out of it and say, "Let's go see the patient." We walk into the room,
and in the first bed sits a petite, middle-aged woman with very
short silvery-gray hair, brown eyes, tanned skin, a friendly smile,
wearing large-framed Warby Parker glasses. I walk over to the
bedside and shake her right hand. "I'm Dr. Thompson. I'm in
charge of this team."

She says, "Hello, so nice to meet you." Even as I am shaking
her hand, I am also examining her arm—the swelling, the streaks
of red, and the ink markings where the residents outlined the
extent of the erythema. And then I just can't help myself—I
immediately jump in with a barrage of questions.

"When was your surgery?"

"Eight months ago."

"Who was your surgeon?"

"Dr. Margrit Bretzke, at Abbott."

"Who is your oncologist?"

"Dr. Michaela Tsai." Wow, I know her. She was a fellow
resident in my internal medicine program, exact same year as
me. She married a guy named John Crowley also in our class
who went on to become a hospitalist while she completed her

heme/onc fellowship. This also explains why she is on a general medicine service and not our inpatient oncology service. She's not "their" patient; she hasn't been followed here at the university. Nope, indeed, she is all mine.

I just keep right on going. "Sentinel nodes or axillary lymph node dissection?"

"Full dissection," she replies. "Twenty-eight nodes in total were taken."

"When did the edema develop?"

"About three months ago." She goes on to describe her complicated home regimen of compression sleeves, one for day and one for nighttime, as well as a pump device she wears for one hour a day and ongoing physical therapy appointments.

Well, I can tell by just this much of the story and the length of her hair that she's also had chemo and radiation, which are both likely contributing factors in this entire ordeal. I need no more information at this point. I do see the small abrasion on her right thumb, and think, *Wow, I have much bigger scratches on my right wrist at this very moment from playing with my cat Harvey.* He has a favorite toy, a stuffed fish on the end of a pole with a bungee cord attaching it. It's basically a more complicated game of fetch, but he loves it. He will leap into the air after this stupid thing and land with it in his mouth or even flip over on his back and start to pummel it. I got too close, just days ago, trying to grab the pole and start the game all over again when his back claws scratched my right forearm. I find myself glancing down at my own arm even as I am standing in front of the patient, listening to her. I'm wearing a short-sleeved dress today; it's a very warm day for early June. I still have faintly visible ropy cords from the axillary web syndrome, but I don't see any redness or swelling. Just the healing cat scratch. *I've got to be more careful.*

I snap myself out of it once again and ask her, "How are you feeling now?"

She says, "Much better than last night!"

Ah yes, there's nothing quite like bacteremia to make you feel like total crap. I mention to her that we'll get our lymphedema specialists to come by. I then hear from her, "My family is hosting my daughter's high school graduation open house tomorrow afternoon at our home in Highland Park, Saint Paul." Her teenage daughter is sitting to the left side of the bed in the visitor chair and nods, gives us a weak smile. My heart truly sinks. After all this patient's been through, certainly much more than me, and now this, another setback, more days in the hospital, another major family event possibly missed. I immediately think of ways to help her. Could she maybe get out of the hospital even for a couple of hours? Highland Park is nearby. Cefazolin is dosed q 8; she has eight hours in between doses of IV medication. Could that be enough time to visit? We'll have to see, there must be something we can do.

"Well, you sure landed on the right internal medicine service," I say. It just came flying out of my mouth. I didn't intend to say it; I was more thinking out loud. My team is mystified by this comment. The patient nods and smiles but also looks a tad bit puzzled. So I try a cover-up: "These residents and students are simply the A team." She laughs then goes on to tell me she also works at the university and has roles in teaching and research. "Really! What do you do?" I ask. She's a professor of immunology, a PhD scientist. We chat a bit about that.

The team and I leave the bedside, and we all stand outside the door. My mind is still blowing, but I don't have much to add to their assessment and plan, so I try to simply pick up the pieces, take a deep breath, and say, "Great job. Now let's head over to 5B."

We finish rounds. It takes about another hour and a half to see all the patients and get plans set for the day. Later, we are back in the team room. After reviewing Epic charts for a while, I tell the residents, "I'm going to my office for a bit and will return later." Instead, I head right back over to 5A and into her room again.

I sit down; her daughter is no longer present. I had wanted to find out honestly what time this graduation open house was, and with that in mind, I could possibly come up with a plan to let her out of the hospital for a few hours in between doses of IV antibiotics. However, now as we are talking, I am contemplating once again, *Do I open up about this, about my situation? How much do I share? Is this relevant at all? Is it helpful in any way, or am I just blabbing about unnecessary details for my own personal benefit?*

However, just before I came in, I also read in her chart that she is part of a rowing team called Dragon Divas, made up exclusively of breast cancer survivors, as well as a community advocacy group. That's one thing I have not yet experienced— being part of a group or a network specifically devoted to coping with this disease. I've felt so blessed, I guess, with my safety net of friends from choir, school, and church that I didn't yet feel the need to specifically seek out something of that nature. On the other hand, I do admit I feel the strong urge at times to talk to other women who have been through this. And I get that. I can totally see why. So realizing there is just something about cancer and feeling the need to connect, I decide, what the heck.

"I just want you to know that I appreciate what you've been through the past year. I'm a breast cancer survivor as well."

She responds, "Really!" and says now she realizes why I made that comment earlier. She sits up, immediately interested. "You look so young. How did you find it?"

I told her, "Self-exam. I hadn't even had a mammogram yet."

"Incredible! When was your surgery?"

I mention, "April 26."

"Wow! So this is all really recent for you. You are *back at work?*"

I explain that with my follow-up results, nodes negative, and favorable Oncotype, I did not need to have chemotherapy.

"That's huge."

"Indeed," I agree. I mention that I will be taking tamoxifen and then feel incredibly guilty that I have not even started it as of yet. (After this week! I swear!) I also lean forward, extend my arm, and show her the cords. "I have axillary web syndrome but no lymphedema, at least not as of yet."

She groans and says, "I honestly hope you never have to deal with this." We get to chat a bit more, and she asks, "Who are your doctors?"

I tell her, "First, Todd Tuttle, now Anne Blaes." She knows who they are. We discuss the nuances of seeking care within your own system and from your own colleagues. I mention, "Half the benefit is being on campus here for appointments and lab draws and such!"

She agrees, saying, "I had radiation treatment from Dr. Kathryn Dusenberry at the university for exactly that same reason."

I tell her, "I know Dr. Michaela Tsai from residency. She's fantastic." Overall, it has been a very good conversation. I get the sense that she values the transparency, and I think, if I were in her shoes, I would very much appreciate knowing that the doctor in charge of my care understands what I am going through. And at the end of the day, in all likelihood, I will probably not see her again after this rotation on Maroon. What's the harm in a little sharing after all?

And I decide I am definitely going to figure out a way for her to be at that open house on Saturday. Later that afternoon, I tell her bedside nurse, Annie, about our plans to let her return home for a bit to attend her daughter's graduation celebration. She agrees and thinks this is a great idea. But leaving the hospital just after 6:00 p.m. while driving home, I get a panicky text from my senior resident.

"Dr. Thompson, sorry to bother you, but the charge nurse on 5A just talked with Annie and now is saying that our patient must be officially discharged tomorrow, then report back through the ER to be reassessed or readmitted for IV antibiotics. She wants to speak with you."

I see the text and just have to laugh. I knew this would be the case. I pick up my phone and dial 5A and ask to speak with the charge. I get put on hold for a minute, then connect with a very energetic and insistent RN. "We just don't allow this. We don't do this," she says. "There is no such thing as allowing a patient to leave the hospital on a pass." She adds, "If the patient is that stable, just discharge her!"

I explain, "But the problem is, we need lymphedema therapists to see her, and they won't do an assessment until forty-eight hours after starting antibiotics." Also, per guidelines, we need to see that follow-up blood cultures are negative before switching to oral. I say, "It's really just a question of timing. The patient looks great otherwise. I don't see the problem here." This RN really gives me an earful, and I say politely, "Okay, just tell me what to do. I'll document a note, I'll discharge and readmit same day, whatever it takes."

She tells me, "You must call the patient placement manager in the morning."

I say, "I will do just that." We're locking horns, just a bit. Later, Annie apologizes to my resident, saying, "I didn't mean to cause any trouble."

The next morning, a Saturday, I dial Fairview Direct and ask to speak to the patient placement manager. I am connected with Stephanie, and I say, Hi, I'm Dr. Thompson. I'm the attending on Maroon 2 this weekend.

"I'm sorry to hear that!" she says. It's funny, we do have a local reputation of being one of the toughest inpatient services to manage; I appreciate the nod of sympathy. I explain to her the entire situation and what we are trying to accomplish. She listens intently, not saying anything for some time, and then states, "I'm just going to pretend I didn't hear about this."

"What?" I ask.

She says, "I'll keep her bed assignment. Just tell her to quietly go and come back, and nobody will be the wiser."

I say, "Got it. And thank you very much."

Now, later during rounds, I am so glad Annie is again her bedside nurse for today. She's on my side, she'll keep quiet about this, I am fairly certain. I walk confidently onto 5A and tell her, "Yes, we discussed this at length with patient placement. It's all fine." A new charge is up at the desk, but I avoid any possible confrontation. Ask me no questions; I tell you no lies. Instead, when we walk into the patient's room, as the team interviews her, I am writing on the whiteboard, a communication hub for every hospitalized patient since 2011. I scribe: "Kim is going to be visiting with her family between 2:00 and 5:00 p.m. on Saturday, June 18. Any questions, please page the attending Dr. Thompson, 899-8286."

My patient is absolutely elated. She tells my team, "This means so much to me and my daughter!" She goes on to describe the day's events, the special food they are preparing, the playlist her daughter has chosen for the background music. My residents are so impressed that I have taken on the establishment, so to speak, to make this happen. "Patient-centered care," is all I say in return. It means different things at different times to different people. But as I shake the patient's hand before leaving the room, she locks gaze with me and smiles, squeezes my hand even harder, and I smile and nod in return. We connect very deeply on another level, completely unbeknownst to the learners rounding with me that day.

It's been another moment that I will cherish and remember even after finishing that week of attending on Maroon and in the months to come. An example of the instant bond, a sisterhood of sorts among breast cancer survivors, and how that translates into supporting one another through various endeavors and setbacks, big or small. And more importantly, I get to help a fellow survivor attend her daughter's open house and enjoy this meaningful time with family, something all the more significant to me after becoming a cancer survivor myself.

I am glad she wasn't admitted to 7D, after all.

Chapter 9

THE CLINIC PATIENTS

Isn't it ironic, don't you think?
—Alanis Morissette

N ow, as a practicing physician, I certainly realize that breast cancer is the most common malignancy among American women. Everyone has probably heard the statistics: one in eight women (12 percent) will be diagnosed in their lifetime. There are more than 200,000 new cases in the United States per year. There are 2.8 million breast cancer survivors currently living in America. That's a lot of women, a lot of patients, and certainly, I've followed many in my own clinic over time. Why is it, then, that ever since my diagnosis, I seem to be encountering it more and more? Is it a heightened awareness? Was I just not paying as much attention before my own health issue rises up and hits me over the head? But I find it interesting that in just a few short weeks after surgery, I encounter many new situations in which I need to immediately draw upon my own recent experiences in order to help the patient sitting in front of me. Each time I glance heavenward, I sense God is on His throne, looking down at me and laughing—not out of mockery, but saying, "See how I prepared you for this? Are you not a better person, a better doctor for what you went through? And here you thought I was up to no good."

Patient #1

A little too ironic…

The first clinic patient, mid-June, comes to see me for a pre-op, an excisional breast biopsy, the Friday before the Tuesday operation. She's forty-four. Good Lord, my age exactly. She's had a suspicious area developing on her mammogram. She's felt a lump there before as well, I will find out. She thinks that the lump has been the same for "years." I look at the standard pre-op information entered at the start of the note in Epic, and I see that her surgeon is Todd Tuttle. That part is not surprising; the man's busy. I've done many of his pre-ops not just for breast surgery but other cases as well. What *is* surprising, though, is what happens next.

I knock, I enter the room, I shake her hand, and I say, "I'm Dr. Thompson, so nice to meet you." She's casually dressed in jeans and a black T-shirt, with shoulder-length ash-blonde hair, pale blue eyes framed by square-rimmed gray glasses. She initially smiles and introduces herself, shakes my hand, but immediately her face settles back into a frown. She appears quite tense. I think naturally she must be feeling nervous about this. I'm flashing back to the first three weeks in April, when I was wound tight as a spring and so distracted—to the point of driving back home when I meant to drive into to work after dropping off the kids at school or completely forgetting routine scheduled meetings. As I observe her, the tension in her face, the furrowed brow, the clenching of the jaw, I wonder what I can say or do to help this situation. I ask her, "How are you coping with all of this?"

"Well," she blurts out, "I just want this over and done with." She goes on to describe, in a rather heated fashion, that this has been a very long, drawn-out process because of the multiple steps leading up to it—a slightly abnormal screening mammogram, followed by a call back for additional images, then a follow-up appointment with her primary MD, who feels the need to discuss the case in person with the breast imaging team. They decide on the next steps, eventually calling back with a recommendation to see Dr. Tuttle. She then schedules the actual appointment with him, which wasn't easy to achieve, but at that encounter, he recommends proceeding to an excisional biopsy. Then *that* visit is followed by multiple phone calls trying to schedule the actual surgery date and this pre-op within the thirty-day window. And of course, she says, by now her primary-care doc is out, that's why she's seeing me even though we've never met before. She is rambling a bit, staring off into space and goes on to say: "Boy is that Dr. Tuttle sure busy. He's almost impossible to get a hold of, and even just scheduling this operation is now weeks beyond what I had planned it to be."

Then she turns back to me. "Do you know him?" she asks. "Is he any good?" she demands. "I sure had to wait a long time to see him, and get this done!"

I stare back at her blankly, hardly believing what I am hearing. Then I inhale deeply and swallow hard. Where do I begin? "Well," I say, "I happen to know Dr. Tuttle was out all last week, presenting at an academic meeting in China. That might account for some of the scheduling issues." But then I mention the fact that he has an international reputation in the surgical management of breast cancer also speaks volumes to his expertise in this area. After giving her that information, she appears to calm down a bit. I then say, as far as his skill as a surgeon, I've referred many of my own patients to him. *Read: me.* I've seen his handiwork. *Gee, a lot lately.* In my opinion, he's the best. *I wouldn't have it any other way.* She visibly relaxes even more. I even tell her, "I know that the waiting and wondering and worrying about the outcome probably seemed like torture, but it would be better to have an informed decision and a well-thought-out care plan with the very best people on your team, even if it took a bit longer." Slowly, she nods.

I sigh and inwardly think, *Todd owes me for this.* But wait, I owe him much more—I'll let it go. After this intense discussion, we have to move on to the actual *medicine* of the pre-op. She's young and healthy, but does have intermittent asthma. "I've been using my albuterol inhaler a lot, perhaps too much lately. Not sure why. I've had no cold symptoms or seasonal allergies. Could it just be anxiety?" During the physical exam, I carefully listen to her lungs. They are completely clear, no wheezing whatsoever. After observing her, getting a sense of her personality and hearing the above description of events, I do tell her, "I agree, it's probably anxiety." I think back to how I spent the first fifteen minutes after hanging up the phone. *The biopsy is positive for cancer.* I was hyperventilating, literally, until I forced myself to calm down and make the necessary calls to get appointments with surgery and oncology. Anxiety and shortness of breath can most definitely go hand in hand.

At the end of the visit, I again reassure her that she's in very good hands. After she leaves, I think, well, I just defused an angry patient, maybe even helped to avoid a potential phone call to patient relations. More importantly, I think—at least I sincerely hope—that I turned the tide for her being able to once again have trust in the doctors in charge of her care. For the patient's sake, that is the most important outcome of all. My pre-op physical exam? That was almost completely unnecessary, to be honest, for this young and healthy woman who exercises five days a week. It's the emotional connection that will make all the difference for this extremely anxious patient. And once again, I am reminded that I simply never would have been able to help her in the way that I did, had I not just gone through this experience myself.

How did she land on *my* schedule that day? Things that make you go hmm . . .

Patient #2

Who would've thought, it figures . . .

The week following, I am seeing another patient—a sixty-one-year-old male who usually comes in just once a year for a routine physical. He's on medication for acid reflux and cholesterol and has a history of an inner ear condition followed by ENT, but generally speaking, he is in pretty good shape. My nurse, Ann, has just finished rooming him when she comes out and says, "Gee, his blood pressure is sky-high."

I say, "Really? That has never been a problem for him in the past." I tell her, "Let's recheck it once he has a chance to sit for a bit."

I knock and enter the room, and the patient is sitting in the orange-and-gray chair next to the computer desk, arms folded across his chest, tapping his foot, looking extremely tense. I've known this gentleman for almost the entire time I've been on faculty—at least ten years or more of continuity of care. He's usually quite easy-going. I see next to him, on that desk, the dreaded tablet device that we use for check-in. Perhaps something happened during this process, or maybe just the sheer length of that intake questionnaire really got to him. Been there, done that. "How have you been?" I say. "I haven't seen you in a while!"

"I'm really stressed out," he says. "You probably saw my blood pressure. My wife was just diagnosed with breast cancer."

Whoa, I sit down. I remove the tablet sitting in the space between us and set it on top of a linen bin behind me. We're pushing all that aside. "Well, that's a really big deal. Let's talk about it. What stage is she?"

"I don't even know!" he blurts out. "All I know is it's so big they need to give her chemo first to shrink the tumor before they will do surgery!"

I pause. I think, *How much information should I give to him? Will this be helpful at all without me knowing the details of the case? His wife is not my patient.*

"I think that's probably stage 3, then," is what I tell him. "Who is her surgeon? Her oncologist? Is she going to seek care at the university?"

"No, we live five minutes from North Memorial. She's seen an oncologist there, but hasn't chosen a surgeon as of yet. She's only fifty-five! She's in perfect health! No family history!"

"Well," I say after another deep breath, "this is a very common disease. You certainly do not need a family history to consider the diagnosis, but it's also very treatable, even stage 3. The fact that she's healthy is a good thing in terms of outcomes. North Memorial, you say?"

And now I turn to the computer and pull up not Epic but Google Chrome, and I type into the search tab: *Dr. Dana Carlson.* She's a breast surgeon at North Memorial, one that I had researched myself; I had considered her among the top five before I ultimately chose Todd Tuttle. "I have the name of someone she should see." Pretty soon, I am routed to the North Memorial website, where

I find an entry in a physician directory with a photo and a bio. I hit Print and hand him the page. "Dr. Dana Carlson is excellent. I highly recommend her."

He stares for a while at the sheet of paper, then looks back at me. "She's really worried about having surgery. She's afraid she might lose . . . you know . . . the entire breast."

"Yes, you mean a mastectomy," I say. "Mastectomy versus lumpectomy usually depends on the type of tumor and the size. After mastectomy, there are many options. She could choose to have reconstruction or not. Some women opt not to. They just want to avoid unnecessary surgery." My voice trails off for a second. I can't believe I am saying all this. I pause, swallow hard, and begin again. "It's an entirely personal decision. You should both feel supported, whatever you decide. She'll want you to be a part of this as well." Believe me, I know.

Now, he's just staring back at me with a somewhat puzzled expression on his face. Maybe I'm overloading him with too much information. Maybe he's wondering how I seem to know so much about the diagnosis and management of breast cancer. I've been his primary doc for many years. I certainly don't do this very often at all, but, I venture out on a limb here, thinking it may help reassure him. I say, "I am a breast cancer survivor myself. Luckily, mine was caught at an early stage. But I very much appreciate exactly what you two are going through right now."

"Wow, are you doing okay? Thank you for saying that!" is how he responds. I tell him I'm doing just great and have fantastic doctors taking care of me. But immediately I turn the discussion back to his wife; we spend a few more minutes talking about the next steps. "Her chemo regimen will include the one they call the 'red devil.' Do you know what that is?" he asks. Ah, yes, the infamous doxorubicin. They've been reading about the side effects online—vomiting, hair loss. I am now well aware of why his blood pressure has been so elevated as of late.

I do eventually go on to the physical exam and update his health-care maintenance, and at the end of the encounter, he thanks me again, shaking my hand for a very long time and with quite a firm squeeze. It's been a good visit, and I think possibly a good idea, after all, for me to open up about my diagnosis. It seemed to help him, just a bit, for what it's worth.

Four weeks later, the very same patient is on my schedule again—this time for "back pain." I think, *Huh, I've never evaluated back pain in this man before now.* I go into the room, and yes, he's strained his back, in part because he and his son are building a backyard fence. But actually, I will come to find out that he really just made this appointment to be able to talk more about his wife.

"We met Dr. Dana Carlson. We really like her a lot. Thank you for the recommendation." I find out she will have a bilateral mastectomy with immediate reconstruction later this summer after chemotherapy is completed. She's currently almost halfway through the round. She's losing all her hair. He describes to me the elaborate head scarves and colorful hats she's been wearing.

We chat some more, and mostly I just listen. "Therapeutic listening" is the medical term for it. Unlike other times, when a patient is going on and on for a long while and I'm letting them but honestly I'm just thinking about what I should fix for dinner, this time I am more or less riveted. I'm trying to decipher what type of cancer she has, what stage, if it's genetic, or why she is opting for a fairly extensive surgery when I have patients in my clinic who were also stage 3 that were treated conservatively with a lumpectomy. I don't ask this, though. It's her personal decision and I really don't need to know, but I am also reminded of how some women will request a bilateral mastectomy because they think it will somehow reduce the risk of cancer in the opposite breast even when there is no evidence to support that. I can't say this for sure, it is pure speculation, but I have to wonder.

For now, with this particular patient, I am definitely listening intently, nodding, and offering both verbal and nonverbal support. I am also very glad that Dr. Dana Carlson is a good fit for them. After all, I did all this legwork, researching just about every surgical oncologist in the Twin Cities—I might as well have someone else benefit from it! It's been another good visit. At the end, he shakes my hand and again asks me how I am doing. I tell him, "Just great, fabulous. If she ever changes her mind or wants a second opinion, well, I happen to know some fantastic surgeons and oncologists here at the U. I can vouch for them first-hand, my A team." He smiles and nods. "I'm really glad to hear that."

"Go, M Health!" I say. He laughs. I even note, after he leaves the office, that his blood pressure is near normal today.

Patient #3

Life has a funny way, of sneaking up on you,
When everything's okay and everything's all right.

The next patient situation that gives me pause is another pre-op—this time for an endoscopy and biopsies to evaluate a new pancreatic mass in a fifty-eight-year-old otherwise healthy female, followed by potentially another surgery. I review her recent scans. Immediately, I think, *Good God, let's hope this is benign.* Pancreatic cancer is very aggressive, notoriously difficult to treat, although by imaging, it does appear resection might be possible.

But wait, there's more. After I knock and walk into the room, I hear the full story. "I am six weeks post-op from a *bilateral mastectomy* due to high-risk genetics. I had multiple family members diagnosed over the years with cancer, either breast or pancreatic, and I began to worry." She's an RN by training, although in recent years, she's gone into business for herself, selling dietary supplements and fitness books and other health-minded retail items. But given her medical background, seeing all this family history, she sought an opinion from a genetic counselor, and they suggested ordering a panel of tests. She describes, with many similarities to my own experience, the period of extreme anxiety, waiting for weeks on these results, then finding out and immediately thinking of her two children.

Flashback: As a relatively young patient, newly diagnosed with breast cancer, I had the thought (as well as my doctors) that this could potentially be genetic. What a strange conundrum that was. The physician in me needed to know why. Was there possibly another reason for this? Could it be related to something other than pure random chance? At times, I *wanted* one of these genes to turn up mutated, saying, "Aha! That explains it!" But then again, on the other hand, *please no,* a genetic mutation carries big implications for the surgical approach—I really wanted to spare the left!—as well as additional tests, screening for ovarian cancer or more, and more importantly, potential risk for my children.

I met with a genetic counselor, Olivia; and just prior to that appointment, I had unearthed some information about my biological father—that he had prostate cancer at a relatively young age. Since BRCA is associated with both breast cancer and prostate cancer and due to the fact that my cerebral cortex was being bathed in truly mind-altering levels of cortisol and epinephrine at the time, I made the big leap—the immediate assumption that, of course, this was going to be genetic. In a moment of sheer insanity, I opted for genetic testing—and not just BRCA but a panel of seventeen different genetic mutations known as the BreastNext. This is so unlike me. In my own practice, I tend to order fewer tests than my colleagues. I take a minimalist approach; I rely on clinical judgment coupled with close follow-up. But at that moment in time, I am obviously not thinking straight.

Ultimately, after weeks at an outside lab, my BreastNext panel turns up completely negative. What boring follow-up for Olivia— but still, I was very happy to hear back from her, actually getting the call on my mobile literally *moments* before I was wheeled into the OR on that Tuesday, April 26. Thank God I didn't need to convert to a bilateral approach at the very last minute.

But for this patient, sitting in front of me, it turns out differently. "Unfortunately, I have a mutation in PALB2, which increases the risk of both breast and pancreatic cancer. I was referred for a bilateral prophylactic mastectomy." She quotes over a 70 percent chance of developing breast cancer in her lifetime— by some estimates as high as 90 percent. I find this interesting; she's already almost sixty years old and hasn't had anything show up yet on her mammogram. Still, if I were in her shoes, I would be considering the same thing. Reading further, she finds out that the risk of pancreatic cancer is also higher but, per the literature, "not as well defined." And as far as her children are concerned, PALB2 is autosomal dominant; they each have a 50 percent chance of inheriting the same mutation.

"Well, at least I sailed through the operation, and now I've been injecting saline into tissue expanders several times, anticipating reconstruction." She reports everything's gone very well so far but is obviously nervous about the pancreatic mass. We talk about this; I mention the benign appearance on imaging, the relatively small size of it, possible resection, and so on. No point in worrying her unnecessarily, at least for now.

I perform the standard head-to-toe "pre-op physical exam" for this patient who is very fit and healthy, and it is completely normal. Having not much to discuss in terms of any pre-op recommendations, we spend the last few minutes at the very end of the visit chatting about genetic testing in general, how the wonders of sequencing the human genome and gaining a better understanding of cancer biology have led to an explosion of potential screening. However, at the same time, to both of us, it feels a bit like opening Pandora's Box. She says, "I'm considering going back to school and becoming a genetic counselor myself." What an interesting idea. I respond, "Your personal experience with the situation would lend a perspective that would be immensely helpful to your practice, and your patients." It would equip her for those times of delivering the news, good or bad, knowing first-hand the emotional responses that go along with it.

I encourage her to consider it. She says, "You know, I see these very young nursing students—and also young doctors— going straight through training right out of high school or college, acquiring new skills, learning to interact with patients. But I almost think, every one of you should have to go through *something*, some sort of health crisis, or endure a chronic health issue, maybe alongside a family member, in order to fully understand what it's like. It's the only way to become any better at it . . . don't you agree?"

Yes. Indeed.

Later, almost two weeks later, I'm finishing up clinic for the day, and I suddenly remember back to seeing this patient. I cannot help but log in to her chart in the EMR and find out what happened. As it turns out, the biopsy was positive for malignancy—IMPN, or intraductal mucinous papillary neoplasm, with some atypical high-grade features. There are only two entries into the chart after this: one is a phone call to the patient, and the other is a referral to a specialist in Rochester for discussion of a Whipple procedure. Then, nothing.

Reading all that, my heart feels heavy. I pause, and I take a deep breath. Inwardly, I utter a prayer for this patient and her family; it's all I can do, at this moment in time. Then I log out of the EMR and head out the door, leaving most of my progress notes unsigned for tomorrow. For some reason, I really want to get home early and hug my kids.

Patient #4

Life has a funny, funny way of helping you out.

I supervise internal medicine residents every Thursday morning in the primary care clinic. They have continuity clinic scheduled for the full day. During this time, they will see and evaluate a patient first, then come out and present the case to a faculty member. Then together we come up with a plan and go back in the room and explain things to the patient. There are six residents and two preceptors present, so it's a bit random as to who staffs the patient or which ones we will see; however, we get to interact with all of them the entire three years of their IM residency. We come to know each other very well in terms of knowledge base, practice style, and so on.

As it turns out, Thursday is possibly my favorite day of the workweek. I have the privilege of resident clinic in the morning, grand rounds at noon, followed by more leisurely office hours in the afternoon. These IM residents are highly skilled, extremely bright, and very knowledgeable. At one point, Charlie said that it's the residents that are teaching him, not the other way around, and I couldn't agree more. Also, they are just a fun group of young people, so enthusiastic, high energy, and with a great sense of humor. As they progress through their training, it becomes more and more collegial and less a supervisory role.

The primary care clinic at the U has also been for many years, the number-one most requested site for continuity clinic for our incoming interns out of almost a dozen options. At times I have pondered; I truly wonder why. We have a somewhat difficult patient population, after all. We're tertiary care, a transplant center. We often see and evaluate patients with not one, not two, but *three* solid organ transplants—yes, heart, lung, *and* kidney (after the heart/lung transplant meds destroy their renal function) or liver and kidney (after hepatorenal syndrome sets in and the beans never recover). We also have a large population of somewhat rare diseases—typically autoimmune (dermatomyositis with interstitial lung disease has become my new favorite as of late) or malignancy. (What? You haven't heard of Howel-Evans syndrome? What kind of doctor are you?)

So one would think that this patient population, coupled with the ongoing follow-up, in addition to the usual primary care health-care maintenance, might seem a bit overwhelming to young doctors in training. But no, there is something about our clinic, the faculty, the nursing staff, and even the patients that really draws them in. We have a great camaraderie and a love of teaching that seems to trump all that.

Speaking of trump; recently, I'm being taught how to play bridge. It's a complicated game, to say the least. I'm still learning from my mom who belongs to a bridge club in our home town of Milaca, playing once a week, and my brother who is in finance and a card shark and a whiz with numbers. He will count cards and always knows exactly how many trump cards are left and that sort of thing. And the thing about bridge is, it's all in the bidding. You need to bid your own hand, but also you must try to read into your partner's bid, interpret the language even though, of course, it is strictly verboten to use body language or tone of voice or additional verbal cues to help accomplish this. Sometimes, honestly, my discussions with patients remind me very much of bidding.

One Thursday morning, my resident, James, has gone in with a new patient. She's a sixty-year-old woman who is here to establish care. He's already seen her, discussed all things health-related, and performed a physical exam. He's presenting the case to me when he says, "She's refusing any and all cancer screening. Despite my advice, she won't even consider it. Nope, she has totally made up her mind. I even canceled the three orders that were teed up by the rooming staff, including a colonoscopy, Pap smear, and mammogram."

I see this quite often myself. I ask him, "Okay, what is your approach to this?"

He says, "Well, patient autonomy. I try to inform her of the risks and benefits and let her decide."

"Yes, that's all well and good," I say. "That's what they teach you in med school. But here's my take on it. What screening test do you think is more important, most high yield, most relevant right now as a sixty-year-old female who is not sexually active and hasn't been for years?" (I like to give residents lots of leading information when I ask them questions.)

"Well," he says, "cervical cancer is pretty unlikely."

"Yes, I agree, HPV and all that. Do you know," I say, "that even colon cancer is approaching more like a 3:1 ratio, males to females? And typically the age of onset is older for women than men?" (I only know this because of my teaching in a second-year med school course.) He seems surprised to hear that. Then I ask, "What do you think about the mammogram?"

He says, "She's beyond the gray areas of the guidelines. She really should have it done. It's the most common malignancy in her age group."

"Bingo," I say. "Usually, if I can talk a patient into *one* screening test, just one preventive health-type thing, then maybe later on, they will reconsider and agree to the colonoscopy or immunizations." We try not to overwhelm the patients; we approach things one step at a time. That's the beauty of primary care. There is always the opportunity to schedule a follow-up appointment, another time to revisit the discussion. Establishing rapport, that's what it's all about.

So I tell him, "Let's go back in and talk about just the mammogram a little bit more." He says, "Good luck with *that*. I'm fairly certain she's going to say no. She recently had a friend who experienced a false-positive result." *We'll just see*, I think.

I knock and enter the room with James. He sits on the small round stool where the doctor typically sits. The patient is beside the computer desk, in the orange chair, and I pull up another orange chair so the three of us are sitting in a triangulated fashion. The patient smiles and shakes my hand. She's friendly, but I must admit, she does have a certain determined air about her. She's rather tall, with broad shoulders, short and spiky silver-gray hair, round black glasses, and she's wearing a colorful red paisley maxi dress with bright-blue Birkenstock sandals peeking out below the hem.

After a bit of small talk, I mention nonchalantly, "At your age, we do recommend a few routine screening tests. One of them would be a mammogram." (Bid: one diamond.)

Well, she flatly states, "I'm not going there. I had a friend who just had this done. They saw some sort of shadowy area.

She needed a biopsy and had to wait almost a week for the result. That's way too much stress and worry for me." (Bid: one spade.)

"False positives can occur," I say very matter-of-factly, "Here at the Breast Center, we have the new technology of mammography with tomosynthesis. It offers a 3D reconstruction of the breast tissue, with better image quality and fewer false-positive results." (Bid: two diamonds.)

"But I have no family history!" she says. "Nobody has breast cancer, not my mom, or my sisters, or either grandmother."

To this, I reply in a very neutral tone, "Breast cancer is so common, one in eight women, that you really do not need a family history to consider the diagnosis." *Believe me, I know* is what I think but do not say. Instead, I mention, "Breast cancer is by far and away much more common than either colon cancer or cervical cancer in your age group." (Bid: two spades.)

"What if I do have an abnormal result?" she asks. "Then what happens next?"

I go on to describe our breast center, their team of radiologists, surgeons, oncologists, nurses, and the integrated, coordinated, multidisciplinary approach. I say, "If the mammogram result looks suspicious, they will perform additional images, usually an ultrasound, and offer to biopsy it right then and there. You will get answers very soon. And the breast center is located on 2B, just two floors down from where we are sitting right now, in clinic 4B." (Bid: two no-trump.)

She pauses and turns to James, who enthusiastically nods in agreement. *Good job*, I think. *We're tag-teaming here.* She then looks back at me and says, "Oh, all right, I'll do it but ONLY if I can get it done today while I am still here." (Bid: pass.)

I turn to James with a look that says, "Make it so, number one." He pulls up Epic, starts to type the order, and gets out his phone to make a quick call down to 2B. Out loud, I say to her, "You've made the right decision." The patient then turns to James and says, "You know, the reason I am agreeing to this? The real reason I said yes? She just gave me facts, information, and no judgment. She wasn't shaming me or making me feel guilty for not doing this all along." She turns to me with a slight smile. To that, I respond, "I'm just so glad we've been helpful to you. And we'll check the result later today."

James and I leave the room. After the door is shut, we fist-bump. "I can't believe you convinced her to do that!" he says.

"Watch and learn, grasshopper," I say jokingly. But here, once again, at this moment, what I am really thinking is this: *I can only provide all these facts and pieces of information in the most relevant and meaningful fashion because of the road I've been walking down myself.*

It's becoming part of me as a physician; it's now just as ingrained as my medical knowledge, my bedside manner, my communication skills, and so on. It keeps coming back to me. It keeps showing up in so many different situations, not just this patient or the three mentioned previously, but on hospital rounds, in teaching sessions—the list goes on. I am fairly convinced, in the big picture, that this is one of several reasons God allowed this in my life, to begin with.

And in life, just as in the game of bridge, I'm learning; I've got to use strategic bidding to maximize the cards I've been dealt.

Also, as it turns out, ultimately, the patient still wins the bid; her mammogram is negative. I'll just have to convince her at the follow-up appointments to keep playing.

Patient #5

It's the good advice that you just didn't take.

I have a few patients in my panel whom I would honestly consider friends. Usually, it is because we have some connection outside of medicine. One patient, as it turns out, was briefly my roommate in college, sharing an apartment in Roseville just blocks north of Hamline University. She came down from Duluth to the Twin Cities for a three-month summer internship, moving in with me and Jean and Rebecca for that time, then returned to UMD. Years (and I mean *many* years) later, she somehow lands on my schedule for "establish care/routine physical." I walk in the room, and I immediately recognize her: "Tammy! Oh my god! It's Heather!" What a coincidence.

She says, "I thought it might be you. You got married! Your last name is now Thompson Buum!" We spend the next twenty minutes catching up on everything before I realize, oh yeah, maybe I should perform that physical exam. She followed up with me for many years after that before moving out of state; each visit was definitely half social, half medical.

I have several longtime patients who are also physicians at the university. Wow, are those visits hard to keep on track. We commiserate about anything and everything. When Allscripts and later Epic was rolling out, it was all about the EMR and the hellishness and how on God's green earth we were going to make this work. When the new dean of the medical school arrives, we talk about the academic atmosphere and how it might be changing. The emphasis seems to be shifting even though we're all the same group of faculty, the same learners, and the same stakeholders. Later, it's all about the new clinic building, anticipating those changes, how to handle the transition. Immediately after *that*, it's the talk of the health system merger, and what happens next? Is the financial rug being swept out from under us? But despite the generalized fear and trepidation and the angst that accompanies academic medicine, I highly value each of these visits. I look forward to them; I am blessed to have the opportunity. Honestly, it means that much to me—the connections, the camaraderie—that I almost feel guilty for submitting an actual bill for the encounter. It probably benefited me more than them!

Another patient of mine, Jane, I've followed for well over a decade. She's a musician. She plays flute professionally and also gives lessons on the instrument. I'm also a soprano in the Oratorio Society of Minnesota; we have our usual musicians in the orchestra for many years now—about half are professional, half semiprofessional. Around seven or eight years ago, I notice a lady on stage during a dress rehearsal; I am staring at this woman. *How do I know her?* I eventually recognize Jane as my patient. She is sitting in the orchestra at Ted Mann Concert Hall, playing her flute. It is sometimes hard for me to identify my patients out of context, such as at the mall or dining out in a local restaurant. But now, I make the connection. Jane is very talented, I observe—the pure notes, the breathless tone, the beautiful fluttering. I make a mental note to mention this next time I see her in clinic.

Well, this I do, and we immediately bond. She asks me, "How did you hear about Oratorio? What are your impressions of the new director, Matt Mehaffey? What do you think of the repertoire for next year?" We have great conversations. This goes on for several years. Every time I see her, we talk about music much more than medicine, and then at the end of the visit, I find I will need to check labs or refill medication or something else to make it seem official.

I am looking ahead at my schedule the day before when I see Jane has an appointment on Friday, September 9, at 4:00 p.m. I haven't seen her in a while; certainly not since my cancer diagnosis. I smile; this brightens my day. I am very much looking forward to the visit. The next afternoon, I walk into the room, and the very first thing she says to me is "Wow! You sure are skinny. Is everything okay?"

Now, this is true. I've lost a bit of weight throughout this ordeal. The first five pounds was probably just stress, poor appetite, not eating. Then the next five pounds, post-op. The five pounds after that (I researched this extensively), possibly a side effect of tamoxifen. It's got to be. Everything else is the same, my eating, the exercise; but I can't seem to move the needle back up past 110. I honestly don't know how to react to her comment. At the same time, I think how observant she is—she obviously knows me *that well*. Wow! I tell her, "As it turns out, I had my own health issue this past spring, but I am fine now. It's all good."

She looks at me intently and says slowly, "Well, I *guess* I'm glad to be hearing that." She watches me sit down on the small round stool in front of the computer. I can tell she's wondering what on earth I am talking about, but it's hard to know, hard for me to decide at times how much information to disclose. My husband has been chastising me as of late for revealing too much about myself or my medical diagnosis and thinks I am shoving my book down other people's throats by asking them to read and comment. So I clam up, about that anyway, for the time being.

I say, "How have you been? Did you have a nice summer?"

"Great," she says. And immediately, her next question of me: "Are you considering Oratorio again for next season? I know you told me last year, you were going to sit out for a while, that you were just too busy, but I didn't think that was such a good idea."

"Ha," I say, "funny you should mention that. I basically did a 180 on that one!" I tell her that I even rejoined Oratorio for the optional summer chorus, something I've never done before. I usually only sing during the regular season.

"Oh! That's so great! I couldn't be there for summer chorus. My family was on vacation that week. What did you perform?"

I am immediately transported back to Mendelssohn's *Elijah*. With a big smile on my face, I tell her all about it. "The chorus sounded fantastic for a non-auditioned group, perhaps because many of us had sung it before. The orchestra was great, although I sure missed seeing you with your flute on stage! And the soloists, wow, we had a ringer in the role of Elijah, a rising star with the Metropolitan Opera, whose voice was like butter." I mention that the performance ended with an immediate standing ovation, something that doesn't happen all that often. She's smiling, then lets out a little gasp, then clasps her hands on her chest in front of her, hearing all this. And I tell her, "I'm coming back for the regular season as well. We have only two concerts next year instead of three, and one of them is at Ted Mann right here on campus, and they both happen to be Friday evening performances, which work much better with my schedule. It's all falling into place. I hope to be seeing you there!"

"Wonderful!" she says and then asks, "What made you change your mind?"

Again, deep breath, pause. How much of this do I disclose?

"Well, I mentioned that health issue this past spring," I say. She nods rigorously. "It really made me realize how important music was to me. The true healing power of it. I just couldn't let it go. After the health crisis, I decided, life is too short. I want to spend my time doing the things that truly matter, that keep me whole and keep me sane. It was definitely the right decision. That *Elijah* performance, it meant so much to me. It was as though I was getting my life back on so many levels."

In the middle of this, she's nodding. Then suddenly her eyes well up with tears, and she actually starts to cry. I see a box of tissues on the desk in front of me behind the computer; I grab it and hand it to her. "Damn menopause!" she says. I laugh, and I tell her, "I can relate, I am now in the same boat."

She dabs at her eyes. "I've heard this from so many of my music students." She goes on to tell me of her experiences over the years, teaching the flute and hearing similar stories. "I've had a student who is struggling in some other area, whether it's work or school or life or health or family or even an addiction, and music is the one thing in their lives which allows for catharsis, a release. It sustains them, just as it sustains you." I am getting a lump in my throat, listening to all this as well.

Eventually, after a few more minutes of conversation, I gently turn the discussion back toward her health issues. Yes, she has questions about menopause, and also, I need to recheck her thyroid levels after I adjusted the dose of her medication. We have been talking for so long, I decide to just skip the physical exam, bring her back in a couple of weeks (she's overdue for a "full physical" anyway), and then I can review the labs at that appointment. She gladly agrees. "I'll schedule this on my way out. I'm so happy you are back!" We shake hands as I stand up to leave.

Later, I will think, *Back to what? Back to work? Back to Oratorio? Back to life?* I hope, in a sense, that it's all of the above.

Also later, I am finishing up her progress note in Epic. I click on the button that allows me to bill for the total time spent with the patient instead of the individual elements of an office visit—the history, the physical exam and so on. In doing so, the EMR will remind me, "Counseling and coordination of care must comprise at least 50 percent of the encounter."

Whose counseling? I wonder. Which one of us is the patient, and which one is the physician? Who is recovering from illness, and who is the healer?

I would say, the two are getting very difficult to separate. Both/and. *All of the above.*

Chapter 10

SUMMERTIME AND THE LIVING AIN'T EASY

She acts like summer and walks like rain,
Reminds me that there's time to change, hey, hey.
—Train, "Drops of Jupiter"

There are probably dozens of books out there describing how a health crisis can change a family dynamic, in particular how it might affect young children and how to deal with it. I certainly could have availed myself of these resources or involved a therapist, a family counselor, a support group, or the youth pastor at my church. However, I decide that, since everything to do with my cancer diagnosis occurred right before summer break, I would use that summer and the extra time to observe both Sam and Lydia, see how they were coping with things, and how this may or may not change their outlook on life before investing hundreds of dollars in self-help books or psychologist fees. To this day, I am still not sure if this was the right or wrong approach, but it's what I thought made sense. And since Monday is the one day when I don't have patients scheduled in clinic, I can often work from home or take the day off as a vacation day, even at the last minute, without having to reschedule patients. I took full advantage of this, June through August of 2016.

Sam and Lydia are almost three years apart; and when I look at them, physically and emotionally and personality-wise, it is as though Paul and I split the gene pool and assigned different sexes. Sam, the firstborn, who is almost twelve, is so much like me. At times, it's like looking in a mirror. He has pale-blue eyes, sandy-blonde hair, and a slender build. He very much resembles me in the looks category. Since he's firstborn, as was I, he also has many of the same personality traits. On the positive side, that means he's been described in the past as extroverted, confident, having leadership qualities that teachers comment on during conferences or in his report card. Other children, at school, in our neighborhood, at church, look up to him and seem drawn to him. On the negative side, when younger, all this (and his fan club, his entourage) means he's also been described as a talker, a bit of a class clown, enjoying constant interaction; he often got into trouble in the classroom because he would be laughing or joking around with his friends when he was supposed to be paying attention. Now that he's older, those personality traits have evolved. He's a bit more quiet and introspective but still has strong ideas and opinions. He can sometimes come across as being willful, stubborn, once in a while a bit argumentative, never wanting to admit he's wrong or might have made a mistake, in particular when it comes to Paul. I'm not sure if it's the testosterone or just two alpha males in the same house or what, but boy, the two of them can sure lock horns from time to time!

Speaking of testosterone, this summer is also notable for a major transformation in regard to Sam—yes, he's growing up, definitely entering adolescence. This seems to me to be happening much, much too early! Maybe I need an endocrine consult for precocious puberty! But there's no denying it—he finally surpasses me in height, his skin and hair are getting oily, and his voice starts changing. I notice just a bit of moodiness setting in, at times; the surly groans when I try to get him out of bed in the morning, the eye-rolling when I ask him to take out the garbage, the gruff response to his sister's questions. I sincerely hope that this is not a personality change due to the increased stress around the house last spring; however, observing him and thinking it through, I start to believe it's all testosterone-related. Also, Sam is now taking that "extroversion" mentioned above to a whole new level. He wants to dye his hair *blue*, and honestly, the only potential time to do this is summer. There are rules at his school regarding uniforms and general appearance, hair included. So at the store one day, I find a temporary hair-coloring kit—Blue Burst—and I give in; I let him do it. Once again, I am reminded of myself at age thirteen, experimenting with hair color but not quite this drastic, going from a dark blonde to a lighter blonde with that go-to product of the '80s, Sun-In.

Lydia, on the other hand, is a Buum through and through. With dark hair, olive skin, hazel eyes, she's quite a beauty. She'll break hearts someday, and sadly, when I look at her, it seems I really can't take credit for any of it. When the two of us are together, I don't think anyone would automatically assume—from a physical standpoint—we are a mother and daughter; the genes in the looks category seem mostly to come from Paul. And even beyond that, she's one of the most artistically gifted, creative, craft-driven children I've ever met. She will take an entire afternoon to sculpt animals out of scrap paper and tape and then fashion an "apartment building" for them out of spent paper towel rolls and old cardboard boxes from deliveries to our home. I will look at this, and then I will see Paul's architectural drawings on the foyer table, and I think, *Wow, the apple doesn't fall far from the tree.*

The other personality trait she gets from Paul: she's a worrier. Yes, even at age nine, when the biggest concerns during summer break should be trying to schedule a park playdate or checking the weather forecast to determine the local library versus the nearby pool for an outing. She tends to perseverate on many things. At the start of the school year, for example, she was very worried about the discipline system in the classroom, a stoplight: red, yellow, green. She wants to know how a student moves from green to yellow to red, what exact behaviors define each, and what would happen back at home if she does. We talk it over, and then I try to ease her mind by telling her about my grade school teachers moving my desk to the front of the room to get me to stop talking to my friends or assigning lunch hour detention for passing notes in class. At one point, I drove my second-grade teacher so crazy, the school administrators moved me up to third grade mid-October just to see if that would help; these days, I would have probably been placed on Ritalin. But knowing Lydia and her attention to following rules, none of these issues would *ever* occur for her.

She also tends to perseverate on physical symptoms as well. For example, after hearing my Mom relay a particularly colorful story regarding an episode of food poisoning from a local Mexican restaurant, she became very alarmed about the possibility of it happening to her. It even reached the point where, that evening, we are out at our local coffee shop, and I allow her to eat too much, having a scoop of ice cream on top our usual artisan cheese tray, and she develops a slight stomachache. She's then convinced she's going to spend the next several days in the john and is, in fact, rushing in and out of the ladies' room at the coffee shop half a dozen or more times while we are trying to listen to jazz, fearful she might be getting "sick."

Once, she and our summer nanny were playing nail salon and giving each other home manicures. Later, she read on the bottle of nail polish remover: "Warning: toxic if ingested." I came home from work and found her sitting at the kitchen table, distraught, convinced she was dying from acetone poisoning because she licked her fingers after eating some popcorn and thought she might have tasted it. I sat down across from her at the table, trying over and over again to reassure her, telling her that the nail polish remover had evaporated long before the snack. "You probably smelled it rather than ingested it. You'll be fine. You do not have acetone poisoning. You would have to drink the entire bottle for this to occur, and I'm a doctor for God's sake! I know some toxicology! You should not be worrying about this!"

Sam wandered into the room, leaning up against the kitchen counter, listening to the two of us go on. He's a very perceptive boy, quite mature for his age. Regarding this acetone poisoning, I will soon find out he's also been trying to convince Lydia all afternoon that she'll be okay, as well. At which point I said, exasperated, "Lydia, you sure have your dad's personality through and through! The worry, the fear, the anxiety! You are your father's child!" At that point, Sam looked at Lydia, then back at me, and simply said, "It has begun."

God, let's hope not. I would prefer not to deal with generalized anxiety disorder in *yet another* family member. Personally, I think I would rather have breast cancer, honestly, than to experience irrational fear at every turn in response to the smallest of everyday events. I then start to wonder if my health situation has also been adding fuel to the fire. Thinking, what have I done here? Now she's probably trying to go to sleep every night, wondering if *I* will somehow get sick or my cancer will come back or if *she* will end up getting breast cancer someday, as she's already asked me about several times. What can I do? How can I make this any better?

Over the coming days, I think about it, and I decide, I will help them cope in the only way I really know how. I start to relay to both of my children, all summer long, at every turn, the many positive things that have happened since my cancer diagnosis. And many of them as a direct result of it. I keep telling them story after story, several of which I have written about in my first book.. In fact, I even let Sam read parts of it, the chapters that detail many of the amazing happenings, the incredible coincidences, the profound circumstances surrounding my diagnosis, and all the support I received as a result of it. Although since some of the subject areas are a little sensitive, I decide Lydia might be a bit too young for it. Someday, though . . .

So instead, one evening, I am in Lydia's room, tucking her in for the night, and I'm trying to make this point sink in. I say boldly, "I thank God every day for this, for what's happening to me. I'm actually glad that I have breast cancer."

"What?" she says. "That's crazy! Why would you be *glad* to have cancer!"

"Well," I say, "if it wasn't for breast cancer, I would not have the following [and yes, I list them all off]: stronger friendships with many women, including Jodie, Amanda, Karin, Rachel; a mentor-now-father-figure in Charlie Moldow; and a new friend and colleague in Todd Tuttle. I have a novel appreciation for all aspects of my work by experiencing the health-care system myself first-hand, including the ability to connect with my patients and walk them through tough situations. Suddenly discovering a passion for writing, both academic and otherwise, resulting in (all in a span of just a few months) a memoir, several excerpts, a case report, an editorial, and three works in progress—a Med Ed Portal submission, a patient-centered observation manuscript, and a collaborative paper on mentoring in medicine."

And in all things, the most important outcome was learning how to *trust*. Trusting in my friends, family, colleagues, mentors to be there for me, and also trusting in God. "Trust in the Lord with all your heart, and lean not on your own understanding. In all your ways, submit to Him and He will make your paths straight." That was my Grandma Jeanette's favorite verse, Proverbs 3:5–6. She often wrote it on the inside of cards and books that she gave to me. In fact, I tell Lydia on the morning of surgery, "My friend Amanda sent me a link to a song as a text message to encourage me. How perfect is that!" Music is such a big part of my life. I practically have my own personal soundtrack going through my mind at any given moment. Even before getting her text, I loved this song; I so enjoy hearing Lauren Daigle's big and rich voice, one of my favorite artists, the Adele of contemporary Christian music. She's even crossed over to the pop music stations in the Twin Cities as of late with her hit "You Say." This particular song sent by Amanda, though, also summarizes beautifully what I'm trying to convey and how I cope: "Trust in You." I've played this tune while driving in the car many times so that we can start to appreciate the meaning behind the lyrics.

> When you don't move the mountains, I'm needing you to move
> When you don't part the waters, I wish I could walk through
> When you don't give the answers, as I cry out to you,
> I will trust in You!
> You are my strength and comfort, you are my steady hand
> You are my firm foundation, the rock on which I stand
> Your ways are always higher, your plans are always good
> There's not a place I'll go, you've not already stood
> I will trust in You!

And that is truly the most important outcome, the most important life lesson of all.

Later, nearing the end of summer, Lydia seems to have processed everything a bit more, and she is less anxious overall. Although as I noted from the very beginning of all this, she's been quite curious about me and my physical state, my physical well-being. She had even asked me before surgery if she could feel my breast lump. After I thought about it for a while, I finally did let her, as it was quite superficial. At one o'clock as they say, just above my bra line and easily palpable, even to a nine-year-old girl. She made a face at the time, halfway between a frown and an expression of disgust, which made me laugh. Later, after surgery, she became curious about my incision and the drain, checking the output, the amount, the color, and so on. Now, many months later, she is a bit obsessed with my scar. She wants to see it and check on it from time to time, monitoring the progress from what she called a "bloody gash" to a bright pink to now fading to a more flesh-colored, pink-rimmed line with a ropy and shiny and slightly raised border. When the axillary web syndrome appeared, she also monitored the cording on my forearm near every day. Since it was summer, it was much more visible, quite obvious in the short sleeves and sundresses. I can't help but wonder, from time to time, if all this would have a positive or negative long-term effect on any emerging self-image, as far as Lydia is concerned.

Then as we are approaching the start of the school year, I am once again reminded of the importance of body image and accepting physical changes. I realize I need to shop online for school uniforms. I ask Lydia if her jumpers and polo shirts still fit from last year or if she needs anything new or different for the school-day wardrobe when she says, "I should really start wearing a bra."

What? At first, I think, *No way, this is much too soon, and you don't really need one.* Then I have this thought pop into my head: *Well, technically, I wouldn't need one, either.*

I ponder that for a minute. Huh, the irony here. But instead, I ask her gently, "Why do you think that? Is there a reason you want to start wearing a bra?" She replies, "There is something official in the student policy manual, and all the girls in my class were talking about it." Admittedly, I never bothered to read said policy manual. I go to my desk, rummage around, and find it and turn to that section. Sure enough, it says that girls in fifth grade and up must wear either a camisole or a bra underneath their school uniform.

So I tell her, "Okay, next time I'm out shopping, I will look around." That weekend, I'm at my favorite department store, the one where I found the athletic bras with the removable pads, and proceeded to purchase about twenty of them. Then I wander into the girls' section to take a look at undergarments. I find several bras that are padded, even pushup, underwire. I am thinking, *No way*, when suddenly I spot a pack of five colorful "bras" that are really just modified camisole tank tops, only shorter. No pads, no lace or bows or ribbon, just a nice soft cotton bandeau in bright pastels with contrasting trim. Perfect.

Once I get home, I present the package to Lydia, and she is very pleased with my purchase. She loves the colors and the soft fabric and proceeds to hug me and thank me several times. She wants to go into her room to try one on; she seems happy and excited to have this new addition to her wardrobe. I come in, sit down on her bed, and watch with a little sadness in my heart this rite of passage into womanhood that seems to be coming just way too early.

As I am taking all this in, I am also thinking once again that I am glad I chose not to reconstruct. Maybe, just maybe, this will have some small benefit to Lydia someday as she is growing up so fast, soon to be entering adolescence. It's too early to tell, but perhaps the fact that there is at least one woman in this house who chooses not to let her self-image or her body confidence be defined by a cup size—who knows, that might just have a positive impact, a side benefit of sorts, one that I honestly didn't even consider up until this very moment in time.

Another life lesson for both my children and me. Perhaps there are even more valuable things that cancer can teach us right now or further down the road—if we can keep our hearts and minds open to receiving it.

She listens like spring, and she talks like June,
hey, hey . . .

Chapter 11

THE WAITING IS THE HARDEST PART

Just wait, and it will come.
—Blues Traveler

With the Moldow family in Idaho for three weeks, I'm feeling a little bit lost, alone, on my own for almost the entire month of August. This month, and marching on into September and beyond, also turns out to be a period of intense waiting for me. Waiting, wondering, idling, standing by, biding time, sitting tight, pining away, holding on, lingering, all of which for me is at the very least annoying, at times downright painful.

I am not the most patient person, to begin with. Waiting patiently, persevering in that sense, is not my strong suit. Although when I consider my career, the many years it takes to train as a physician, the delayed gratification and all that, one would think that at my age, I would finally be getting better at it. What am I waiting on right now? Well, as is typical in the world of academic medicine, it's grants and publications. We all have to get used to this, the long waits, as well as papering the walls of our offices with rejection letters. It's just part and parcel. It's par for the course. This is nothing new. At this point in time, I am waiting on the innovations grant from the medical school to support curriculum changes in my second-year course, a case report, a workshop submission. And of course, there's the book. I've excerpted two chapters and sent them to literary journals designed for physicians as writers; I've also submitted the entire manuscript to two local presses—after three very speedy rejection letters from prominent New York City publishing houses. For all these projects, it's been the writing that has been the easy part; the waiting, after submission, much harder.

It starts to remind me, actually, of my pregnancies. The many months' wait, the anticipation, the yearning for the day when motherhood is not just an abstract concept but a reality. This was especially true for Lydia, who was a week overdue. At that point, I'm already on maternity leave, predicting—since I went just a bit early with Sam—that I might go early with baby number 2. It turns out I was mistaken. Also, our nanny of over two years had just left, transitioning to graduate school, so rather than find a new child care provider right away, I am already at home on leave with Sam, who is almost three. I spend those days power-walking around Lake Como, pushing him in the stroller, eating extremely spicy food, trying anything to jump-start my labor. I almost couldn't stand it any longer when, *boom*, water breaks at 2:00 a.m. on a Sunday and Miss Lydia arrives at six that morning. She's eight pounds, eleven ounces, looking quite puffy and bruised. She's all wrinkly from too much time spent in the amniotic fluid and has numerous bruises from the ultrafast labor, barely having time to sneak in the epidural. In the newborn nursery, the pediatrician who is rounding that weekend stops by, looks at her, turns to me, and says, "Was she a little past dates?"

So now, I am in another pregnant pause, as it were. There's not a thing I can do to speed up the process. Jogging and spicy food won't work. I start to question the wisdom of submitting a manuscript to an academic press during the summer months when, at any university, everything slows down, so many standing committee meetings are cancelled, and half of our faculty are up north at the cabin or even summering in the Hamptons. And without Charlie around during August, I have fewer people to talk to, to vent about the book, the long wait, the delays. Not many colleagues even know I have this sort of publication in the hopper. And my family? They've grown so tired of hearing about the book, it's almost verboten around the house. My kids created a "swear jar" to this end with a label on it that reads, "Book." Any time I mention the book, I will have a put a quarter in the swear jar. Soon, I will either declare bankruptcy or fund the kid's college this way; it is filling up far more rapidly than the ones I made for the kids.

But during this time, I am still getting updates from Charlie about every three days—at least he still has email and internet access in this remote and pristine location! He's enjoying the vacation, the perfect weather, the lack of humidity and mosquitoes, the time with family. Although for the second update, I get an email on a Monday morning, saying he had to go to the ER over the weekend because he threw out his back. They order a CT. It shows a disc bulge at L1-2; now he's returned to the cabin but can barely move, and asking, "If you are not too busy, could you please talk to Jim Langland about sending a medrol dose pack to the local pharmacy?"

I'm very sympathetic to the back pain, but as far as the prescription, I just have to laugh. Langland is out of town again. Man, that guy travels a lot. I need to start to emulate his approach. But I'm also his practice partner, his "buddy," as our medical director calls it. I help cover him when he's gone, and we also share the same RN, Tony, who assists both of us in patient care tasks. Well, "assist" is not the right term. "Runs the entire show" would be more accurate. And also, this is a Monday, that one day I don't have patients scheduled, so I am working from home. I am sitting at my kitchen table, reading my tablet, and instead, I just pick up my phone and dial the number on the screen and start to ramble off the prescription and Charlie's name and date of birth and my name and my Minnesota medical license number.

I type back a response: "I've phoned this in myself. Go start it right away. Stretching will help too. And I guess we cannot blame this on either Merkel Cell Carcinoma or our favorite M Health surgeons."

He replies: "No, it is the fact that I am being held together via duct tape and wire."

I laugh, and then mention: "Just don't ask me to phone in any Percocet."

He responds: "The ER offered opioids in abandon and were simply shocked when I declined." Again, I chuckle, having the same aversion to narcotics myself. Post-op, I was sent home with thirty tablets of oxycodone; I still have twenty-eight of them left. I guess I am keeping them around in case I slip and fall on my run around the lake or roll my ankle, playing basketball with Sam.

The Medrol dose pack works; he's much better in the coming days. But later, just as the waiting is really starting to get to me, I think it starts getting to Charlie, as well. He starts sending me these short snippets of email, very cryptic in nature, but alluding to this fact.

Subject: Book

Text: It seems as if it were a total washout you would have heard by now.

Subject: Book proposal

Text: maybe this editor is a very slow reader?

Subject: Going crazy

Text: Could they possibly take any longer??

As things progress, it now reminds me less of pregnancy and childbirth and more of dating. Pregnancy generally has a defined outcome at the end; dating, not so much. And at my age, after having two kids, then a mastectomy, and until very recently these funny-looking cords growing down my right arm, well, let's just say that would be a challenge, to say the least. I'm feeling very much past my prime. These things all take their toll. Imagine if I'm single and I have to put all of this physical description listed above into an online dating profile. Oh, I'm sure the queries would just come flying in! Perish the thought!

Yes, the book proposal starts to feel very much like dating. I must really be a spinster now; I've been rejected by these three big handsome "men." Now I'll settle for anybody, even what one published author calls "the haven of all unprofitable books, the academic press." And although I am getting *some* email correspondence from the local publishers, they only reply to my initial outreach, nothing sent directly to me. They are few and far between and also very cryptic in nature. I cannot tell if they are positive or negative or if they could possibly indicate any interest whatsoever. I am trying to read between the lines. I am feeling desperate; I am being strung along. Just like in college. As in:

June 23: I email the assistant to the editor three weeks after hitting Send just to confirm that they actually received it, both the paper and the electronic version. I ask if there is anything missing from the initial submission that I can provide. Reply:

> Dear Heather:
>
> I do have your hard copy submission here. Did you email the materials as well? I will make sure the editor sees the electronic files as well. We've been getting so many submissions lately. I apologize for not replying earlier. Best regards.

July 12: Since most publishers want to be alerted of multiple submissions, I email them, saying I've submitted two chapters as standalone essays for review at academic and literary journals. In doing this, I actually am trying to entice them here; I'm showing a little leg. I mention a publication like this, a chapter excerpt of sorts, would serve as a good advertisement for the book later on. I'm "building a platform" as they say in the business. I ask if the Google link is still working. Reply:

> Hi Heather,
>
> Yes, I was able to print off a copy of the entire manuscript, and it is currently with the editor. We should have everything at this point, but will definitely let you know if we are in need of anything else.

August 11: I start an email again, letting them know that as of August 6, the manuscript is complete. I've even settled on a title. The word count is just over seventy-five thousand, which seems like a very good length for a first-time effort. I say I am hoping to find out where things are at in the review process. Then I start to wonder, *Should I be playing hard-to-get? Tell them I am playing the field?* Maybe I should mention I have submitted simultaneously to another publisher in a creative memoir writing contest, just to pique their interest. Nothing like the attention of another man to fire up one man's emotions. But I decide against that and simply hit Send.

Nothing. No reply.

August 26: I decide to let them know that I am working on a sequel. Yes, it's crazy, but after a several-week lapse, a hiatus, I grow a bit antsy. I start to really miss writing, the therapeutic aspects of it. In another moment of sheer insanity (considering I can't even get book 1 past an acquiring editor), I open up another Google doc and start book 2, a continuation of the story. I surmise, they may want to know about this. It may actually appeal to a publisher, in case they fear I am a big risk, just a one-off, writing only this one memoir and then immediately reverting back to writing progress notes, discharge summaries, and prescriptions. Fueled by something: Competitiveness? Insecurity? Feeling the need to prove myself? I send another email, attaching the first three chapters as a sampling, a preview. At least this time I get a reply.

> Hi Heather, thanks for following up on this. And I'm so sorry that it has taken a while to get you a response. We will be meeting on Monday for a good while to consider several submissions, and we will be certain to get back to you next week on where things stand.

I read this with some excitement then forward to Charlie: What could it mean? His equally cryptic response was "I think they are saying this is not bad for the Jews . . . Welcome to the tribe."

Then a week passes, then another. It's eighteen days after this supposed Monday morning meeting, and still, I have heard nothing. After that rush of positive energy, I am falling back into deep despair, almost a clinical depression. Unlike rejection of a paper on residency clinic or course innovation or some other academic, educational endeavor, this book is so intensely personal that it feels like an outright rejection of *me*. This is high risk, emotionally. I have never been in this situation before. I start to feel a bit off physically as well—fatigue, headache, nausea, as well as tons of heartburn. Everything I eat gives me terrible reflux. This is eating me up inside literally and figuratively. I start to think, *If I do finally hear back and it's another no, I'll be stuck in the loo, vomiting copious amounts of bilious fluid. I will be calling in sick to work.*

I have lunch with Charlie and Gay on a Friday, mid-September. They had just returned from Idaho last week, and it's so good to see both of them back, but I am definitely not in the brightest of moods. I have a hard time doing anything but complain, and then I feel even more terrible because this is so unlike me. Where is the optimism, the sense of humor, the energy? One of my older patients always calls me Little Miss Sunshine. I feel as though there is nothing but clouds and rain lately. The next day is a Saturday, and I look ahead at my calendar and think, *Thank God. Next week, I will start another week of inpatient attending.* The complicated patients, the team rounds, the teaching, the whirlwind pace—this will actually do me some good. It should be a welcome distraction. It will occupy pretty much all my time, my brainpower, and my thoughts, even energy and emotions, for the span of seven days. It almost reminds me of back in early April, when I was in the throes of panic and anxiety from the cancer diagnosis. I did so much better at the office than at home, ironically, in terms of coping.

Once again, perfect timing. My profession, my work as a physician, will save me from myself.

There's no such thing as a failure who keeps trying;
Coasting to the bottom is the only disgrace.

Chapter 12

TICKET TO RYDE

Golf is a game for everyone, not just the talented few.
—Harvey Penick

I really only watch or follow, with any regularity, two professional sports: NFL football and PGA golf. Although lately, with Sam into basketball, I'm trying to pay more attention to that as well—taking in college hoops, as well as NBA games. Jim Langland has twice given me tickets to a Gopher Men's Basketball game, complete with passes to the Club Lounge for snacks and beverages. We thoroughly enjoyed these outings. We have also attended three Timberwolves games at Target Center, including a win against the Lakers, featuring LeBron James as their star player. In our neighborhood in St. Paul, we have several small private colleges nearby—Hamline, Macalester, St. Thomas, Northwestern. I'm a Hamline grad, and so three years ago, I started to take Sam to Hamline basketball games at Hutton Arena, which is just a mile south of our house. But quickly realizing that the Tommies were the team to watch, we also ventured down past Summit Avenue to the beautiful, modern Anderson Athletic Center at St. Thomas and watched them beat up on the Pipers. It turns out they even won the 2016 NCAA Division III Men's Basketball title, the second time in the last six years. I then signed Sam up for Coach Johnny Tauer's basketball camps at St. Thomas that summer following, thinking, *Well, the man must know what he's doing, obviously.* The camps were very much a reflection of that, a positive experience. Sam even recognized many of the players and learned from them as now camp coaches.

But for me, as far as any *active* sports participation, I decided to take up golf in 1995 as a second-year medical student. It's a bit of a cliché, the association between doctors and golf; but actually, in my large group practice in the primary care clinic, I am one of only two physicians who play with any regularity. Mid- to late 1990s, my learning of the game was timed perfectly with the rise and peak of Tiger Woods. His amazing talent and ability were truly awe-inspiring. When we were first dating, Paul and I watched at local bars and restaurants the unbelievable Tiger Slam in 2000–2001, winning all four professional major championships in a row. In 2009, after his image was shattered that Thanksgiving night following the car accident outside his home, I was glued to the television and news reports for days and weeks after, watching in despair his free fall from grace. Tiger, the most dominant player the game has ever seen, almost completely unraveled. It took him another four years to come back and win a tour event in 2013. Eventually, he claimed another major victory at the Masters in 2019, earning his fifth green jacket; golf history in the making.

But time marches on. Many new players arrive on the scene, alongside some of the old greats. Phil Mickelson became my new go-to PGA pro as a real gentleman and an amazing talent, although it's always a bit strange for me watching his left-handed swing. I also appreciate the new talent, the young guns in the form of Rickie Fowler, Jordan Spieth, Dustin Johnson, and Rory McIlroy. However, other than watching the majors and other tour events on television, I had never actually been to a PGA tournament nor seen or interacted with any of the players in person.

Thirteen years ago, when Paul and I were newly married and house hunting for our first home, Paul got two tickets to the PGA Championship at Hazeltine National in Chaska, gifted to him by a colleague at work. I had clinic patients scheduled that day, so he took his friend John, his former roommate and golf partner, instead of me. At one point, early evening, I had left work to meet our real estate agent and walk through a house in the

Falcon Heights neighborhood, near the University of Minnesota campus, in between the state fairgrounds and the Como Park area. I fell in love with this quaint 1941 brick cottage. Given it was a terrible market at the time (every house selling in a matter of days with multiple bids), I tried desperately to call Paul and see whether he could meet me and walk through it together that very same night or tomorrow morning, not remembering that he was at a PGA event and couldn't even have his cell phone with him. I think I left around twelve voice-mail messages before finally realizing what the problem might be.

Fast-forward to spring of 2016. One big disappointment with the timing of my surgery is that it occurred right at the start of the golf season; the diagnosis came via a phone call the same week as I was watching the Masters. I immediately thought, *There goes my swing for some time. Dang it, why couldn't this have happened in November or December or January, when there is really nothing to do in Minnesota but hunker down and watch football?* Also, the April 26 date of surgery was only five days before the Liberty Golf Classic on May 1. This is a tournament that serves as a fundraiser for my kids' school. Every year, we participate. I solicit donations from friends, family, and local businesses, and I look forward to playing the actual event. It's a very nice golf course with a program and luncheon served afterward. Sadly, on that particular day, I had my sister in law Kasey play instead of me as a "ringer," along with my dad, my brother, and Paul. Wouldn't you know, their foursome won the entire tournament! Unfortunately, I had to stay behind and volunteer to help organize the room for the lunch and program. It was literally post-op day 5. I still had a *drain in place* underneath my ruffled top, and I thought, *Gee, I probably shouldn't be lifting these chairs and moving these heavy tables around and everything else—but oh well.*

But then, on the flip side, I tried to remain positive. I reasoned I could still be back for the end of the season; I really like fall golf—playing in the cooler temps, taking in colorful leaves. That is a great time of year to play, although it starts to get tricky with the prospect of losing your ball among the fallen leaves. Also, come fall, there is—again hosted at Hazeltine—a big event, the Ryder Cup, being held the week of September 26. Match play, very exciting, United States versus Europe. I remember back to

Paul and John attending the PGA Championship at the very same course, and I ask him, "Do you think you could get tickets to Ryder Cup? Maybe utilize your connection at work? That would really be something to look forward to!" I bug him about this late summer until he says, "I just don't see this guy anymore. I haven't been able to make anything happen." So I stop pestering him about it. Sigh. I guess we are not going to the Ryder Cup after all.

At this point, it's early September, and I'm just getting back into golf. After completing physical therapy for my axillary web syndrome in July, I've been to the driving range a number of times and played an official round for the first time in August. My swing is right back to where it was before all this happened; I'm amazed at how muscle memory works in that regard. Then on Friday, September 9, I come home from work, and I take in the mail. In it, there is a thick white business-size envelope. The return address reads, "Minnesota Section PGA," with the official blue-and-gold emblem beside it.

What on earth is this? I am thinking. I feel the envelope. It's heavy. Something more than just a letter must be inside. I open it up, and the first thing I see is "The 41st Ryder Cup Spectator Guide." I slide it out from the envelope, and two tickets to the Ryder Cup fall out from inside this brochure onto the table, complete with elastic lanyards. I pick them up and stare at them, mouth agape. Then I see a triple-folded white piece of paper also inside the envelope, and I slide it out and open it up. On the official Minnesota Section PGA letterhead, it says:

> Paul and Heather,
>
> Thank you for your support of the Liberty Golf Classic last spring! Enclosed are 2 International Pavilion tickets for the 41st Ryder Cup Match, good for September 29, 2016.
>
> Sincerely,
> Darren DeYoung

Tournament Director (and Liberty
parent)

What? I can hardly believe I am seeing this. I show them to
Paul excitedly; at first, he is not even sure they are actual tickets.
He keeps looking at the two passes hanging on the lanyard and
flipping them over to look at the bar code on the back before he
decides, "Yes, it's the real deal."

Sam is in sixth grade this year at Liberty. We've attended the
golf fundraiser for this entire time—that's actually eight years
counting kindergarten and preschool—and *never* have we gotten
anything close in return for our participation, other than a few
door prizes, such as a gift card to a pizza place. What an amazing
coincidence. What a blessing. I bet this Darren DeYoung has no
idea what it means to me, with my recent cancer diagnosis, my
temporary setback, trying to get back to playing golf myself, and
yes, even wanting to get out there and enjoy a PGA event, the
spirited Ryder Cup—which I honestly thought was never going
to happen.

Golf is a strange game. It's almost impossible to master it or
even just continue to improve unless you devote tons of time to
it. But then, every once in a great while, it pays you back. I have
never had a hole in one, but I holed out in Scottsdale, Arizona,
March of 2012—on my fortieth birthday. In my hand is a 5 wood.
I am a bit over 130 yards out. I pause, seek out the target, the pin
with the black-and-white-checkered flag. I take a practice swing,
lining up just a bit left. Then I begin the backswing, pause at the
top, rotate my torso, and give it all I've got. The ball sails through
the air, perfect arch, then lands near the front of the elevated
green, and rolls, and suddenly disappears. I can't see it anymore.
I didn't know what happened, honestly. I just assumed it rolled
off the back edge of the tiny green. Then from the cart, Paul says,
"Hey, I think you should go take a look. It may have dropped in
the hole!"

Upon hearing this, I sling the 3 wood under my right
arm and start to make a determined march across the fairway
toward the elevated green. With each step, I am growing more
and more excited. My heart rate is speeding up. My palms are
sweating. I can't move fast enough, one foot in front of the other,

arms pumping, speed walking the entire 130 yards to that hole. I thought breaking into a run might look strange. I climb up the edge of the elevation, past the bunker, scaling the small hill in record time. Once there, on the flat surface of the green, I stride on toward the pin, staring intently at that 4.25-inch diameter round dark space.

I am now directly over the hole, and I bend over, peering down, shading my eyes from the intense Arizona sun to see within it. And lo and behold, there is my white dimpled ball. It's a Noodle, not all that fancy or expensive as far as golf equipment goes, but one of my personal favorites. It has three large specks of grassy dirt on it, just above the insignia.

I let out a serious yell—a whoop!—and overhead a hawk lets out a cry in response. Both of these sounds echo throughout the canyon in this beautiful Arizona desert expanse. They reverberate back. At this point, Paul and my friend Jodie and her husband, Joe, are all approaching the green with excitement, knowing there is going to be something to really celebrate here after all.

Well, opening that envelope and seeing those tickets to the Ryder Cup, it was almost as exciting as experiencing the hole-out. It also reminds me of how much the game of golf *will* pay you back—if you just keep at it and patiently wait for the opportunity.

Chapter 13

THE (ALMOST OVERLOOKED) FOLLOW-UP APPOINTMENT

> Medicine is a science of uncertainty and
> an art of probability.
> —Sir William Osler

In preparation for inpatient attending, I am looking at both my Google calendar and also the on-call schedule known as Amion. I cross-check Epic to verify dates and to make sure my clinic patients are actually cancelled that week. After I confirm that everything is in order, I look back at my calendar, and I see that I have an oncology appointment, 4:30 p.m., Monday, September 12. OMG! After becoming so wrapped up in everything else going on, I suddenly realize, I almost forgot my own three-month checkup with Dr. Anne Blaes, my oncologist, and this appointment is right around the corner.

I spend the next few days trying to remember what she told me the follow-up might be from the last visit at the end of May. I can barely recall. Was it going to be MRI or mammogram? How often? Did she mention checking blood tests, a metabolic panel being on tamoxifen? I honestly can't come up with anything, and here I am, a physician myself. I start to think, *How do patients with no medical training keep track of all this?*

But then I start to worry, to dread this just a little bit. I don't want any labs. I don't want any scans. Can't I just keep doing breast self-exams on the left? After all, given everything that occurred back in April, apparently my own self-exam is better than a routine mammogram, at least equivalent to an ultrasound, and quite possibly even better than an MRI. And now, I must say, the exam is just that much easier.

I have lost the cyclical breast pain entirely. Well, obviously, not having a cycle since Baltimore in May! Welcome to menopause! I've also lost much of the general bumpiness I used to appreciate while checking for this. And I don't know if it's weight loss or tamoxifen effect or what, but I'm quite a bit smaller, even on the *non-operative* side, which is extremely depressing, to say the least. I didn't have much to begin with, but still, my left breast is about half its original size. So I go online and find many reports from other women on tamoxifen, saying the same thing—regression, "shrinkage," to borrow the Seinfeld term. My new go-to lingerie, the athletic bra with removable pads—sadly, I now need the extra padding on *both* sides to achieve any sort of a silhouette in clothing. Every morning, I will get dressed, pulling the athletic bra over my head, thinking, *This is all so fake.* Then I suddenly stop and say to myself, "Well, so is a breast mound! What's the damn difference!"

Okay, well, back to the follow-up. If I can actually see and appreciate all these changes, depressing as it may be, still, at least it appears the tamoxifen is actually doing something. As far as side effects, the hot flashes that were fairly severe midsummer are actually starting to lessen up a bit. Maybe it's the changing weather, cooler fall temps, or I think I'm adapting, adjusting to the new hormonal balance. I am mulling this over in my mind because I know Anne will be asking me about all this, come Monday afternoon.

Even though I somewhat "dread" the appointment—after all, who in their right mind wants to contemplate all over again the ramifications of having a cancer diagnosis?—still, at the same time, I am looking forward to seeing Dr. Blaes. I want her opinion on all this—my symptoms, possible side effects. I need her expertise, her experience. I also have so much to tell her—my axillary web syndrome is gone, vanished, after just four PT sessions in July! She'll be glad to hear that. I'm also thinking, I should really bring her a gift, something to let her know how much I appreciate the excellent care I am getting. Then ironically, I get home from work on that Friday before. My daughter Lydia presents to me a grocery bag of fresh produce from the neighbor's garden. Vicky actually sent me a text earlier that day, saying, "We can't possibly eat this all ourselves. I'm sending some over!" I unpack this bag, first the ripe tomatoes, then the zucchini and the acorn squash, then lastly, near the bottom, there is another plastic bag folded over. I open it and find at least a dozen good-sized beets.

I laugh and think, *Well, it's about time for Anne to try my grandmother's famous pickled beet recipe.* I had even written about this in my first book. Tony, Charlie, and Todd each got a jar from me early on as a way of expressing my appreciation, but given a rather busy schedule, I hadn't been to the farmer's market in a couple of weeks. Then lo and behold, beets show up at my door. As it turns out, if I just write about these things, they seem to somehow miraculously *happen*—just like the tickets to the Ryder Cup that came in the mail last week! Maybe my writing has magical powers? Hey, what *else* should I put into this book? I win the lottery, get promoted to full professor, then reopen the primary care clinic in a new building with twenty-one exam rooms and three lavish team spaces! Oh wait, that's exactly what we had in the Phillips Wangensteen Building. How about an entirely new medical school building located where the old Masonic Cancer Center once stood, right next to the hospital? And build a new clinic, with the PCC as the one and only teaching clinic housed within it. That way, we're closest to the action since I know for a fact we have the most medical students and residents working alongside us at any given time. Maybe, just maybe, I have the Breast Center and Oncology clinics relocate there too. More convenient for *me*, after all, to be located right next to my docs. Dream on!

But I know I will have to make the eight-minute walk instead or ride the shuttle from the hospital to the front door of the brand-new, ultramodern Clinics and Surgery Center at M Health. I will yet again have to navigate that building as a patient, including the electronic-tablet-device-driven check-in, the locator badge system, and the open waiting area that is outside the Masonic Cancer Clinic. I find myself contemplating strange ideas, such as putting my hair up in a ponytail or wearing my glasses instead of my usual contact lenses so that people don't recognize me.

On Sunday afternoon, I enter my own chart in Epic and clean up the med list ahead of time, discontinuing the Oxycodone prescription and also the Lisinopril, which gave me a nagging cough. Thankfully, Candesartan does not. Thinking about that, I wonder if my blood pressure will be okay. I check it with my home cuff and get 128/83, then 115/75, which is good. It's usually much higher at an office visit, though. I can't seem to reverse that phenomenon.

Monday morning, I drop off the kids at school, then spend the better part of my early day working on a presentation—a board review session for the upcoming Minnesota Chapter American College of Physicians meeting. At 2:00 p.m., I head over to the Medicine Education office for a meeting with several faculty who are organizing a primary care teaching workshop in the fall. At 4:00, I leave, and I head over to the Clinics and Surgery Center, deciding to walk instead of ride the shuttle; it's a beautiful fall day, cool and crisp and sunny, perfect weather. University of Minnesota students are out and about in droves, strolling around or riding bikes all over campus. It's the start of the fall semester, lots of activity going on. I walk through the quad dormitory complex as a shortcut to the CSC and pass an outdoor volleyball game, young men shooting hoops, and students sitting around on a blanket, talking or listening to music blaring from their phones.

I walk into the CSC building, take an immediate left, then climb the winding staircase that leads from the first floor to the second floor, right outside clinic 2B, the Breast Center. Once I arrive, I see that the open lobby is much less crowded than I recall during the first follow-up visit. It's nearly empty. There are only a few patients and family members scattered throughout, sitting on the mid-century modern furniture. At first, I think that is good. Then I start to worry. I question, I fear, *Is this because we are losing clinical volume? Are the oncology patients dissatisfied with the new clinic space, the new arrangements? Could they be leaving and going elsewhere?* I hope this is just a random occurrence.

I present my badge to the clinic coordinator at the podium stand and say, "I'm here to see Dr. Blaes." She looks at the badge. I'm just using it as an ID and to show her my name and correct spelling of it; but maybe because it also says, "Doctor," she asks, "You *do* have an actual appointment with her, don't you?"

I say, "Yes, I believe it's the last appointment of the day, the four-thirty slot."

She gets me checked in, and I am handed the locator badge and then told to find a seat anywhere nearby. It's a few minutes' waiting, and once again, no magazines or anything to read. I'm tired of staring at screens. I've been on my computer most of the day, so rather than get out my phone or my tablet, I just sit there, watching the other patients in the waiting area, as well as the nurses and clinic coordinators and other staff milling about. I take in the scene, and again, I observe some of the typical features, the bald heads, the headscarves, and the face mask in place. I also notice, across the lobby, an area under construction. Apparently, they are installing two new lab draw areas for oncology patients so that they don't have to report to the main lab on the first floor and wait in a crowded waiting area with people all around them, many of them ill, coughing and sneezing and whatnot, potentially spreading infection. I think to myself, *Hmm, this building is only a few months old, and here we are already tearing down walls, installing new functional spaces?* Maybe they should have thought of that in the original design. Believe me, we've considered taking a sledgehammer to the wall between the docs and the nurses in clinic 4B.

I finally get called back to the vital-signs area, and the initial blood pressure is 140/90. A good deal higher than at home, and I mention this to the nurse, who says, "Don't worry, we see this all the time. Nobody in their right mind wants to be here. We can recheck it."

I chuckle, and I say, "I can understand that, somewhat." I'm placed in a room, and after a few more minutes, there's a knock and in walks Dr. Blaes.

"Hi there! I haven't seen you in a while! How have you been?" She's smiling, her ice-blue eyes twinkling. She shakes my hand and sits down on the stool in front of the computer.

I tell her, "Great, I feel fabulous. Back to running, back to golf. I even went to spin class today over the noon hour with my colleague Jim Langland, the bicycling enthusiast."

She asks, "How do you find the time to do that? I've got to figure that out myself."

I go on to mention, "Emotionally, I'm also in a much better place," and I comment on the amazing support I've been getting from friends, family, and colleagues.

"That is so good to hear!" she says.

Her next question is "How is your arm?" I am wearing a sleeveless top. It's a warm day for early September. I extend the right arm, show her how the cords have completely regressed, nothing even visible now, and I demonstrate the full range of motion as well. She comments, once again, on how dramatic the cording was initially. I went on to tell her about the case report, on my own axillary web syndrome, complete with photos. She tilts her head to the side, raises her eyebrows, and says, "I thought you were kidding about that!"

"Oh no," I say, "We wrote it up. It's sitting right now with the editor at the *American Journal of Medicine*! We'll see if it gets accepted!" She has a good laugh upon hearing this.

Next, we discuss tamoxifen. I mention the fact that I haven't had a period since May. She says, "Wow, well, don't throw everything out too soon. You may just be irregular for some time." I then describe the hot flashes, which were fairly severe, mid-July to mid-August. They seem to be lessening now, nothing unbearable, and they don't wake me up at night anymore, which is a good thing. I haven't really noticed any other side effects other than, potentially, my weight—I mention my online reading, that 26 percent experience weight loss, per up to date. On the scale today, it's 107 pounds. A couple pounds less than 109 back in May. I tell her, "I am eating normally, calorie-wise. Yes, I've been exercising but no more than previous." She's not too worried about it. She says it's levelled off; it's stable, as long as it's not continuing to drop. Then we both joke about the coming winter and likely some weight *gain* that might go along with that.

The discussion turns toward the follow-up. I ask her, "What about the imaging we discussed last spring? Every six-month MRI alternating with a mammogram?" Inwardly, I think, *God let's hope not.* I've seen my own MRI reports (times *two*), the extreme density, the difficulty interpreting the results. I really don't relish the idea of going through the loud and confining scanner once a year, then waiting two to three days for the result, then worrying that they are going to find some sort of ill-defined shadow to biopsy, and then wait several days after *that* for a potential answer.

She then says, "I think we should revert back to once yearly mammograms, with tomosynthesis, or 3D reconstruction. It is a very good study. I usually reserve the six-month MRI for high-risk patients; with your low Oncotype score, and the changes you have noticed already being on tamoxifen, I personally feel you are a low risk even though your age is right on the cusp."

I respond, "That would be great! I'm really a minimalist!" I was dreading ordering any labs or scans or anything that would not be medically necessary or was not truly evidence-based. We are in total agreement on that one. This was the best possible piece of news for me at that appointment. I'm certainly willing to stay on tamoxifen, come hell or high water, if all I need is an annual mammo!

We go on to chat a bit more. I then present to her, in a blue-and-red-plaid gift bag, the homemade pickled beets. She lifts the jar out from the sack. I ask, "Have you ever tried pickled beets?"

"No!" She says. "How interesting! I'm looking forward to it. But really, you shouldn't have!"

And I tell her, "Well, people seem to either love them or hate them. Don't feel obligated to finish the jar if they are just not your 'thing.'" And as for the gift, I say, "It's my way of saying thank you for all the support over the past few months." She smiles and tucks the jar back into the gift bag with the tissue paper surrounding it.

Lastly, I mention, "I have one more question for you, but it's completely unrelated to medicine." (Well, sort of.) I go on to tell her about my book. I say I've written a memoir of sorts about my experiences with breast cancer, and she's mentioned in it quite a bit. I tell her, "It's all very positive, a tribute to physicians at the university. I hope that you don't mind if I use your name. It's currently under review at a local press, but don't get me started. It's sure taking a long time for them to get back to me." I even offer to send a few chapters, maybe an excerpt, the ones she's mentioned in, if she wants to see it in context. It may never leave my Google Drive, I say, but regardless, I wanted her to know. I tell her, "The book has a lot of humor in it too. Trying to find the bright spot in dark situations."

At this point, she's pushed her stool back and away from the desk and is sitting there with arms folded across her chest. Her mouth has dropped open slightly. "You wrote a *book*? An entire memoir? In just five months?"

"Yes," I say, I really have no idea how or why, but once the inspiration set in, I just ran with it. "I'd love to see a copy. I'd like to read the entire thing, actually! I think I would really enjoy it." So I tell her, "Yes, I'll send it to you as a Google doc. Check your email." And she says even before reading a single word of it, "Go ahead. You can use my name."

We move on to the physical exam, and she wraps up the appointment by checking the status of refills on the tamoxifen. It's been a great visit. I'm so happy about the follow-up, no imaging again until April—and here I had been dreading this all along. Why? I don't know, but now it feels like another burden has been lifted.

Ironically, Charlie's appointment with his oncologist, the follow-up of a rare type of aggressive skin cancer—Merkel Cell Carcinoma—was also today, *this very same day*. Immediately following my appointment, after I text Paul an update, I send Charlie an email (he doesn't text):

Subject: Great news!
Text: No labs, no scans, Anne says come back in April for a mammogram! Very pleased! H
Charlie's Reply: That makes two of us—off for a celebratory scotch, maybe two.
My reply: Must fill me in on the details! Scotch is not my thing though. Red wine, please!

And so, there it is. We're both doing so very well at this point in time—one with surgery plus tamoxifen, the other surgery plus radiation. For now, it's the best we could possibly hope for.

The next day, I also get an email reply from Anne after I send her the Google doc: "Heather, it was great to see you yesterday. I'm so thrilled with all the things you are doing and how well you are feeling. You go, girl! Inspiring to us all. I look forward to reading the book. Anne."

I read this, and it truly warms my heart. But at the same time, I think, *Really? Inspiring? Me?* I am a bit surprised to read that, honestly. I hold my team of doctors in such high regard; I feel as though it must be the opposite. They are the ones I tend to put on a pedestal. It is they who inspire me, not the other way around.

Then I suddenly realize, I remember, I have so many patients of *my own* that I have followed over the years and truly value those relationships. I marvel at how many of my patients and patient scenarios I am writing into my story. In light of my above reaction, the irony of that is not lost on me. Through my writing, I am coming to realize, yes, it is entirely possible—I can now see that our patients are always teaching and even caring for, and yes, inspiring their doctors to be better physicians and better people as well. In some ways, I knew that all along; but now, my appreciation has risen to a whole new level.

Later that evening, I am looking forward to telling my family in person about the appointment and the good news. I give myself a break from cooking, and we instead head on over to our local neighborhood Chinese restaurant. We sit in our usual corner booth, and Min, the waitress, brings over our standard drink orders without even asking—two Sprites for the kids, two glasses of Chardonnay for the adults. After finishing my usual shrimp in garlic sauce, extra spicy, I open my fortune cookie, and pull out the small white piece of paper:

"You will be rewarded for your efforts within the month."

I show this to Sam excitedly and ask him, "What could this be? You seem to always have the right answer on these." It's like Johnny Carson as Carnac the Magnificent. He can simply press the paper to his forehead and tell me exactly what it means. He reads through it, pauses, and just says, "Your book." Wow, now that shows he's truly paying attention, offering some much-needed encouragement in light of the extremely long wait. I realize, not much gets past Sam these days. And I hope, once again, that he's correct.

Chapter 14

MAROONED, AGAIN

Hospital life, with its byzantine array of moving parts
layered atop the unpredictable rhythms of illness, is a
permanent state of flux.
—Danielle Ofri

The next morning, a Tuesday, I begin another week of inpatient rounding attending on the internal medicine service known as Maroon 1. As usual, I am assigned a team of learners—a senior resident, an intern, and two medical students. I supervise and teach while they follow hospitalized patients, up to twelve, helping to manage their care, come up with the diagnosis and treatment plan, or assisting with bedside procedures. It's a busy week, to be sure. The students quickly find out university patients are complex, a tertiary care population. Rarely is anything straightforward, such as a community-acquired pneumonia or a simple cellulitis. When I have a student presenting, I emphasize this point, saying, "You are actually following three patients rolled into one, which is also why we need three doctors overseeing their care instead of one, but it's all good. It's even better for your own teaching and learning. If you can work up a fever in a patient who is also immune suppressed due to their renal transplant or manage GI bleeding in a patient with an elevated INR and low platelets due to liver disease, imagine how easy this will be in a normal host!"

And working with both the patients and the learners in this capacity is extremely rewarding; I consider inpatient rounds to be one of the best parts of my job. We have the privilege of admitting quite interesting cases, often transfers from outside hospitals where they simply have no idea what is going on, such as, the young woman on infliximab with the recurrent high fevers and pulmonary infiltrates despite broad-spectrum antibiotics. We get to expand the differential to consider all sorts of rare and unusual diagnoses. Gee, I will think, it's probably our old friend Histo, or maybe Blasto, fungal pneumonias with infectious agents endemic to Minnesota. Later on, sure enough, the urine antigen is positive, and the bronchoscopy reveals the oval, narrow-based budding yeast of *Histoplasma capsulatum*.

The medical students and internal medicine residents are also extremely bright and knowledgeable. Ironically, the brand-new third-year student who just took step 1 of the Boards will probably be able to fill out that list of rare pneumonias even faster than a practicing physician. And having a team of enthusiastic young doctors, each of them teaching and helping and supporting one another as they navigate the complex patient care tasks, well, it's very heartening to watch.

I also enjoy teaching them a different aspect of medicine entirely—efficiency: how to get things done, how to expedite patient care tasks in order to advance the care plan and, yes, benefit the patient and family, but also, get out of the hospital at a decent time, avoiding a twelve-hour day every single day. I also try to shorten morning rounds and avoid what I call "helicopter attending." We don't need to see every patient together every day, and this gives the team more time and also the autonomy to make some decisions on their own. From my years as an associate program director, I am acutely aware of how long hours and burnout can affect our residents and also our students. I try to make a point of role modeling efficiency every time I am on service.

Now, most of our young, straight-out-of-residency hospitalists probably think they are the ultimate role model for efficiency; after all, they are like uber residents or a glorified night float. They spend all their time in the hospital. They know the system. They understand how to get things done. But because they *do* spend all their time in the hospital and never set foot in a clinic, I start to realize, interacting with them and signing out patients and whatnot, that there is sometimes a limited understanding of what we as outpatient physicians are capable of in clinic. As in, don't bother fine-tuning that blood pressure regimen or the diabetes management *too* much; it's likely going to be very different once the patient is out of the hospital, at home, eating their normal diet, resuming their usual activities—we will follow up. Or I see that the primary MD has already started that workup for anemia, including iron studies, a peripheral smear. Don't bother repeating all these tests, or going too much farther— leave that up to the clinic doc. And also, since I have clinic literally blocks from the hospital, I reap the benefits of that, and expedite discharge planning by adding them onto my clinic schedule for the following week.

Another point: unlike being just out of residency or only physically located in the hospital, over many years, I have gotten to know more faculty across many different departments, different subspecialties. I recognize who is really good at what and who we can call in a bind for an expert opinion. This connectedness is much easier to achieve when you co-manage patients from the clinic side, for example my patient with lupus who also sees a staff rheumatologist. It comes in very handy when you need to contact that same rheumatologist for help with a different inpatient case. I have found this to be true for surgery, radiology, and even the ER docs as well. After fifteen-plus years and interacting from both worlds, it's just a better working relationship. We tend to trust each other's clinical judgment. I only say all this because it seems as though our mid-career internal medicine faculty, once they hit a certain age, give up inpatient attending altogether because it's too difficult or time-consuming or just doesn't work out with their other academic duties. Residents and students really miss out on some great teaching and mentoring opportunities because of that, *and* the ability to expedite patient care might actually be affected as well. Maybe, *just maybe*, instead, we should try to make it less onerous for older faculty to attend on the wards.

Speaking of which, this time around, I am trying to role-model efficiency yet again when I find out about some major changes made to our inpatient workflow on the Maroon teams. I think to myself, I just finished a week of attending in June, not too long ago. Why is it that every time I am on service, the rules have changed, and everything is different? It seems we can never settle on a system that simply works for all involved. What I am told is that I am now following three "staff only" patients, in addition to the cap of twelve on the resident service. And oh, by the way, when I am on long call, I'll also be taking the triage pages.

What? Triage, at our hospital, is a full-time job in and of itself. You are essentially on call for the entire upper Midwest. I'll get calls from local ERs but also Fargo ND, or northern Wisconsin, or the Duluth area, wanting to discuss cases, possible transfers. Each page is usually a ten-minute discussion, at least. And medicine triage is usually the first point of contact even if the patient really needs ICU level care or would be better served on the inpatient cardiology service or even needs surgical consultation. As a result, the pager goes off *constantly*. But wait, there's more. Also new, there is a triage note template in Epic, with smart phrases and other things I don't fully understand, so then each call should really end with another five to ten minutes of documentation in the EMR. I find out later, our long-call "triage" shift, thankfully, is only noon to 3:00 p.m. At least we get the morning to hopefully finish rounds, but even in that very short window of time, by 3:00 p.m. my pager fills and displays "Memory full," which means over twenty pages were received. Needless to say, I cannot get anything else done during this time, certainly not teaching the students or residents nor staffing any new admits until much later in the day and after I complete all those triage notes. This is really going against my grain, my first principles of efficient use of time.

And not to complain, but the three-staff-only patients also turn out to be a lot of work, quite time-consuming. One is stable, ready for discharge but needs to be sent to an LTAC—long-term acute care facility—and I must complete the very complicated discharge process for this particular transfer, and it takes me almost an hour. Another patient, I have heard from the previous sign out, is, well, rather *difficult*. She asks lots of questions, needs frequent updates throughout the day, and tends to resist our suggestions or have her own ideas about blood pressure or insulin or other medical management. At least, that is how she is presented to me. *Gee,* I think, *great. One of the main reasons I keep doing this inpatient work—teaching and supervising and interacting with students and residents—is starting to get pushed aside, lost in translation.*

This is reminding me, very much, of some of the "newly established" workflows in the primary care clinic after the move to the new Clinics and Surgery Center. When the call center lost staff, the PCC triage calls were suddenly, without warning, transferred to our pool of RNs without any of the other usual patient care duties being transitioned away. As a result, they are accomplishing much less in terms of medication refills, results follow-up, patient MyChart messages, or coordination of care in between office visits. They are essentially on the phones all day long. And the calls can be so random: "What time is my appointment tomorrow?" "What is your fax number?" or even a pharmaceutical rep calling to ask if they can drop off samples. This does not require an RN level of training to handle; these are switchboard calls, essentially. To me, it is truly wasting their time and expertise and taking away from what they enjoy the most—patient care and interacting with their docs.

So when I hear that inpatient triage has been "rolled into" the long call day in addition to a teaching service and following three-staff-only patients, I almost have to laugh, and I send a text message to my nurse Tony. I describe the situation and say, "Hey, don't feel bad. It's not just the nurses that get work piled on—it's the docs too." He texts back right away: "I bet that decision was made by someone who is not a full-time clinician." I chuckle, and I think, *It is, unfortunately, entirely possible.*

But I decide I'll have to wait and give this feedback to the powers that be after I rotate off service. I also hear, thank goodness, that this is all a temporary fix until we can hire more full-time hospitalists. I can suck it up, I guess, for seven days, after all. I'll make it work. And at 3:00 p.m., I am just walking back into the Maroon team room after handing off the triage list to the swing shift doc, saying, "Good luck with *that*," when who do I run into but Justin.

Justin was the right-at-the-end-of-internship, slightly-burned-out first-year medicine resident that I supervised on my last week of inpatient back in June. I had tried everything in my power to make his day a little easier, including using the Epic app on my tablet to expedite rounds, notifying primary MDs that their patients were admitted or discharged, helping to supervise the medical student during a procedure, even using the "scribe" function to sign student notes so that he didn't have to leave *yet another* separate daily progress note or H & P saying the exact same thing. This approach, coupled with my daily jokes on rounds and also his dry wit and great sense of humor, meant that we all got along famously that week. The efficiency even created more time for some sit-down teaching, as well as lunches out at the Campus Club, which seemed to really change the dynamic.

Well, Justin today seems in his element. He's no longer the burned-out intern. He's the big-shot senior resident on the cardiology service. And at least in our program, there is (or should be) a big difference between an intern and a senior. The senior is there to lead the team and to teach as a mini-attending of sorts, and it's a very enjoyable role for most. He's much more relaxed, has a big smile on his face, and he says, "Dr. Thompson! Are you on service *again*? Seems like yesterday we were together!" and he walks on over and leans in and gives me a big hug. He's so much taller than me that he has to stoop over quite a bit, and I laugh and hug him back.

I say, "Hey there! Look at you! How is second year? How's it going on cardiology?"

He says, "Great! I am really enjoying the service and the complex patients, lots of good cases."

I reply, "Glad to hear that! Are they luring you over to the cath lab?"

"No," he says with a laugh, "I like it, but I am still considering GI."

He's from Kansas City, Missouri, famous for barbecue, fountains, jazz, museums, and college basketball. We talked about this last summer; it sounded like a great place for my family to visit. "Have you made that road trip yet?" he asks.

"No," I reply, "but fall break is coming up. Kids are off school in October. We're still considering it!"

We chat a bit more, and now in walks my senior resident with one of the medical students after checking on a new admission down in the ER. Justin turns to my Maroon 1 team and says, "*She* is your attending for this week? Why, you lucky dogs, you."

Well, that truly made my day and put me in a good mood all over again. Here I went from ornery and grumpy regarding the triage pages to upbeat, happy, and so appreciative that I can be a part of a teaching hospital, an academic learning environment, where it's not just about patients—yes, that is very important and, of course, the very reason we exist—but it's also about the little things. Educating students and residents and providing moral support, camaraderie, role modeling, mentoring, and so on. And just as Charlie always comments—it's the residents that are teaching him, not the other way around. At times, it's also the residents mentoring and supporting *me*. Inspiring *me* to keep going despite all the challenges and angst of academic medicine. Not to mention juggling work and family, my health concerns, and everything else.

I wouldn't trade it for the world, not even for a highly paid private practice position or for more predictable hours in administration or a simpler, more manageable, more convenient health system, such as a small suburban clinic where you can park right outside your office space for *free* and don't have to factor in Gopher Football games.

It's a good life.

Oh this has gotta be the good life
This has gotta be the good life
This could really be a good life, good life.
—One Republic

Chapter 15

THE BUDDING AUTHOR(S)

Originality is nothing but judicious imitation. The
most original writers borrowed from one another.
—Voltaire

O n Maroon, many of the patients we admit are transfers out
of the ICU who are now stable enough for the floor. And
considering that our inpatient floor teams admit very
complex, seriously ill tertiary-care patients to a general medicine
unit, well, those that land in our University ICU are quite often
(please pardon the expression) DND—damn near dead. That is,
requiring a ventilator or multiple pressors, battling sepsis, kidneys
failing, complicated by GI bleeding, arrhythmias, and usually,
this is on top of—oh by the way—immunosuppressed status due
to a transplant or chemotherapy or a rare autoimmune disease.
We even have patients on ECMO (extracorporeal membrane
oxygenation) when all else fails and their lungs simply cannot
oxygenate despite maximal ventilator support. This is akin to
being on cardiopulmonary bypass for open heart surgery. Once,
during my clinical-medicine small-group teaching, a second-year
medical student presented (in an impressively succinct fashion)
a patient with lupus, admitted with a fungal pneumonia, then
requiring the ventilator, then ECMO for several days, then back
to vent, trach, eventually the floor, then TCU, then full recovery.

I stare back at this medical student in sheer amazement and say, "So basically, the patient died and came back to life."

She replies, "In summary, yes."

On day 4 of my week of inpatient attending, we accept a patient as a transfer out of the unit who is exactly this type of case. She's a sixty-two-year-old female, Margaret, post lung transplant. She was admitted with pneumonia and septic shock and rapid a fib. She was intubated, had a prolonged ICU stay, and is now finally extubated. The blood pressure is stable, as well as the oxygen levels. But she's a little confused, perhaps due to ICU delirium and the multiple sedating meds it takes to keep a patient on the ventilator. She's also quite tachycardic, heart rate in the 130s. Still, I get a call from the ICU staff, and up to 5B she goes. If there is no ET tube and no levophed, well, she is essentially mine, all mine.

My team presents her case to me. A few questions remain. In particular, the atrial fibrillation with rapid ventricular response (RVR) has been difficult to manage. Her heart rate is in the 120s or higher most of the time even just at rest without any exertion. Margaret was on max-dose metoprolol, and the ICU team just added Diltiazem two days ago to help improve rate control. Also, the residents are appropriately concerned about her mental status, this confusion. Could she have had a small stroke? Infection such as encephalitis? What about subclinical status epilepticus? Do we continue to work this up any further? They report per the chart that she's also had a traumatic brain injury years ago, so we have no idea what her baseline is. After hearing a prolonged summary of her complicated ICU course and tons of data including labs, imaging, and vital signs, *my* brain starts to get a bit traumatized, overloaded. I just say, "Let's go see the patient, and then we'll decide."

We walk into the room. The patient is alert and oriented, actually, but very verbal, constantly talking, sort of rambling on and on. Some of it makes sense, but at times, she becomes quite tangential or interjects a random thought about her medications or how having to consume a dysphagia diet is next to torture: "Have any of you ever *tried* to drink a viscous Diet Coke?" I also notice that Margaret's hands are trembling. They are shaking as she reaches up to smooth her hair away from her eyes or when she is gesturing toward the tray of nectar-thickened liquids sitting in front of her. I then remember, she's had a lung transplant; as I am standing at the bedside, observing her, I have this thought jump into my brain—*calcineurin drug toxicity*. I've followed so many transplant patients over the years, and I recognize that this is how old-school cyclosporine A (CSA) toxicity would present—altered mental status, tremulousness, often hypertension, acute kidney injury as well. On an MRI of the brain, you can see classic white matter changes in this situation. Margaret is on a newer version of CSA, tacrolimus. As it turns out, the Diltiazem started in the ICU for rate control can increase serum drug levels of the tacro. We draw a level; it's 22. Her range should be 8 to 12. Later, I will say to my team jokingly, "That's why they pay me the big bucks as the attending." (Really, not so much as an academic general internist, mind you.) But here's where mid-career attendings might add some value.   I just saved a million-dollar workup for altered mental status based on my clinical experience.

So with this in mind, we hold the drug, and lo and behold, she gets better in the coming days. Her mental status improves; she's still quite talkative, but sharp, and extremely witty, very funny. Margaret regales the team with stories of her many years as a lung-transplant patient, including multiple complications and many hospitalizations, and tells them bluntly, "I have already died four times. I'm like the cat with nine lives. In fact, last week, I thought I was a goner." She goes on to say, "You should have seen the emails my husband sent out to my friends with subject lines such as *'Things don't look good'* or later *'ICU course takes a turn for the worse.'*" She quips, "I think he was starting to write my obituary for the local papers." Then she says, "I needed to call my friends today to let them know I am being discharged and if I could possibly get a ride, and it's like they are hearing from a ghost!" We all chuckle upon hearing this, and I am thinking, what an amazingly strong woman to be able to laugh at the prospect of her own death.

Then she goes on to tell us another incredible story. Because of her transplant meds and even prior to that, being on steroids for many years, Margaret has osteoporosis, very weak and brittle bones. "In my kitchen, at home, alone, a few years back, I took a fall and actually broke my leg doing this, the left femur. I am lying on the floor, experiencing internal hemorrhage, growing weaker by the minute and simply cannot get up. I was just lying there, thinking, 'Well, this is it. I am fading fast. I am a goner.'" Then as it turns out, she's also taking care of her niece's dog, who—just to clarify—has never played a game of fetch with her in his entire life. But at this point, the dog comes trotting into the kitchen with something in his mouth. He leans over and places a rubber ball on her chest. "I used this rubber ball and a strategic throw to knock the kitchen telephone off the cordless cradle and onto the floor, then reach over, and stretching my arm out, I grab it and call 911."

We all marvel at this story. It's pretty amazing, we all agree. She next describes the paramedics arriving at her house who then accidentally let the dog loose into the streets. How ironic. Next, the trip to the hospital and then multiple orthopedic surgeries and the very long rehab that followed. Margaret gestures toward her left leg. "This leg is still a tad shorter than my right, but I get along." Then she says to the entire team but looking back at me, "I am writing a book about my experiences as a patient."

I say, "Well, that's a great idea! I highly recommend doing that! It's very therapeutic; I am doing it myself." And I stop. Did I think that? Did I say that? Me and my big mouth. I don't know if it's the tamoxifen or surviving a cancer diagnosis or what, but it's like I have no frontal lobe these days. No inhibition, I'll just say anything to anyone.

My team all turns to look at me. The patient's face lights up. She smiles, sits forward, immediately interested. "What is the title of your book?" I swallow hard. Oh dear, I didn't intend for it to go this far. But I'm really stuck now. What can I possibly say?

"*Mirth Is God's Medicine.*" I pause and explain, "Yes, it's about doctor becoming patient and all that, but there is a lot of humor in it as well, hence the title."

She literally gasps. "I just got the chills." She goes on to say that having a sense of humor has saved her countless times from falling into a deep despair or even just a bit of frustration given her complicated medical history. And in addition to that, faith is a very big part of her life. She comments, "I don't know how people get through any of this without leaning on God." She turns to the house staff team. "You've got a wonderful example here—a great mentor, I can just tell." I am starting to feel quite embarrassed, to be honest, a bit self-conscious. My face is turning red (or is that the tamoxifen?), so I try and steer the conversation back toward Margaret, the discharge plans, and so on. I ask her how far she's gotten with her book. "I can't type at all," she says. "I needed to download Dragon dictation software, and I'm getting a slow start, but after hearing your story, I am truly inspired to start working on it again."

I respond, "Well then, let's get you out of the hospital. There's important work to be done!"

Later that day, around two in the afternoon, she is waiting for medications to be filled prior to discharge. Her nurse Andrea pages me, saying, "Margaret is asking to speak with you before she leaves." I think, *Okay, what's up?* And I walk back into her room, prepared to answer what I presume are questions about the discharge plans, the medications, the follow-up labs, and so on.

"Sit down." I find a chair in the corner next to the window, and I pull it up. "You look way too young and healthy to have endured any type of health crisis. What happened? I simply must know. If you don't mind sharing, that is."

I pause. Again, I feel somewhat trapped by my own fault. I don't know exactly what to say. But then, well, I think, if this book *does* get published, I am going to have to get used to this after all. Anyone could read it and know what I have gone through. And what I shared before briefly on rounds seems to have resonated so very much with this patient. Do I dare go any further?

"Well, I'm a breast cancer survivor. I had surgery last April."

"Really!" she says. "My sister is a breast cancer survivor! She went on to have surgery, followed by chemotherapy and is doing great, five years out." She then says, "You still look way too young for this. How did you find it?"

"Self-exam," I reply. "And I'm forty-four, actually, not that old but not that young either."

She laughs. "Well! You look *twenty-four* to me, sweetheart. Wait until you get to my age."

This goes on for some while. Margaret is asking me how I could possibly find the time to write a book. I describe the two weeks off after surgery, the downtime in hotels at academic meetings, the late nights and early mornings due to insomnia. I also point to the computer in the room and say, "I'm a lightning-fast typist, thanks to Epic. No Dragon for me." She laughs, and again, she comments on how both humor and faith have helped her endure a number of health crises and face the future with a positive attitude always, no matter what comes her way.

Next: "Tell me about a funny chapter in your book." Well, again, not sure how far to go with this or what might be TMI, but I decide to mention a chapter I recently sent to a literary journal as an excerpt—the MRI Saga. "Enduring an MRI is a really interesting experience—humorous at best, frightening at worst. Especially a breast MRI! The awkward position, the confining space, the loud wailing of the machine." She groans and says, "I know exactly what you are talking about. I've had too many MRIs to count."

I try to turn the discussion back toward the discharge plan. I ask her, "Who do you follow up with here at the university?" And then she mentions Dr. Marshall Hertz as her pulmonologist. I know him pretty well, and I think, what a perfect fit—he also has a sharp wit, a great sense of humor. I mention this to her, and she laughs and agrees. Then I ask, "Who is your primary care doctor?" and she says, "I don't have one. I could sure use a referral."

I reach into my white coat pocket and pull out a business card that says, "University of Minnesota Physicians, Primary Care Clinic, Gold Team Providers." It lists me and Jim Langland as the MDs and Tony Roth as nurse coordinator. I hand it to her, and she reads it over with interest, then looks back at me. "This was meant to be!" she exclaims. "This was God ordained!" And I just have to smile. She then says, "Come over here!" and proceeds to give me a big hug. Man, I am thinking, there sure has been a lot of hugging on this service for even less than one week.

She says, "I want an advanced copy of your book." I tell her, "Well, I could share it with you as a Google doc, but with one caveat—you have to promise to buy a copy once it's out, and I will sign it for posterity's sake. And I want one of yours too."

"Deal!"

Chapter 16

THE DIFFICULT PATIENT

A physician is not angry at the intemperance of
a mad patient, nor does he take it ill to be railed at
by a man in fever.
—Lucius Annaeus Seneca

D ay 1 of Maroon, I am told I am following three-staff-only patients. One of them, Amanda, is a complicated case. She's only forty years old and has type II diabetes for the past ten years. She recently also had hypertension and came in because she developed total body edema, or anasarca, and abnormal kidney function tests. Her creatinine, which was elevated on admission just kept rising, unfortunately, despite fluids and managing the blood pressure and excluding all other causes such as medications or infection. A bit puzzled by this, the team consulted nephrology, and they actually performed a kidney biopsy to discern what exactly was going on. The result was somewhat surprising—severe diabetic nephropathy and with over 70 percent fibrosis—meaning, it was very unlikely her kidneys would recover. Given everything going on, she is approaching dialysis very soon.

The first thing I think is *Ouch, I wouldn't wish diabetes on my worst enemy.* I've said this before. What a complicated disease, often quite difficult to manage even for the brightest, most motivated patients. The long-term complications can include kidney failure, as it appears to be the case for Amanda, as well as neuropathy, retinopathy, cardiovascular disease, or peripheral artery disease, even loss of a limb. A brand-new diagnosis of diabetes often buys the patient five different meds from the very start: one or two oral hypoglycemic agents, a statin for cholesterol, an ACE inhibitor for renal protection or blood pressure, daily aspirin therapy. And oh, by the way, you must now figure out how to use a glucometer and finger stick needles and test strips and check your blood sugar three times a day and learn what to do in the event of a low or high reading. I often think about this and how overwhelming it might be for the patient. There is a reason we have dedicated diabetes educators, RNs by training who go on to specialize in how to help patients manage this disease.

The next thing I hear from the previous attending, who is yet another brand-new hospitalist who just completed residency is that Amanda is rather, how shall we say, *difficult*. He suggests, "I'd round on her right away, first thing in the morning, really early, before even meeting up with the house staff team. That way, you get it out of the way, and some of her questions can get answered. But believe me, you'll spend lots of time, and be prepared to be called back several times throughout the day, particularly after endocrine or nephrology has rounded." Apparently, she has somewhat unique ideas about blood pressure and glucose management, often correlating it with signs or symptoms that don't perfectly make sense, or requesting specific changes that are outside the usual mode of doing things. The hospitalist reports, "I think she's overall just a bit frustrated and fearful of going on dialysis."

Well, again, I can hardly blame her, and I say something to that effect. She's four years younger than me, for God's sake. And the prospect of reporting to a dialysis center three times a week and sitting there during a run for another three- to four-hour interval, not to mention the multiple steps leading up to this, such as deciding on a route for vascular access—this must also be quite overwhelming. But after the hospitalist signs out, I'm also thinking, as far as rounding, getting there any earlier is just not going to work for me since I often drop the kids off at school in the morning. Our wonderful but small start-up classical academy doesn't provide busing as of yet. So I read through the nursing notes, which all say Amanda is not much of a morning person, often prefers sleeping until 10:00–11:00 a.m. and not be disturbed with the vital signs and whatnot until later. I think, perfect. I'm shifting my rounds into late morning or early afternoon, and we'll see how that goes.

My first encounter: I walk into the room, and she is lying in bed, wrapped up in a tan fleece blanket brought from home, with a panda bear stocking cap over her head and a blue plaid sleeping mask over her eyes. It's the triple sign, I note. Three items or three objects that are used to shield the patient from the rest of the medical world. I have seen this in clinic. Often, it's the sunglasses, the earbuds, and the baseball cap; or it's the headphones, the leather jacket, and the fingerless gloves. Some of my older patients, it might be the fedora and the trench coat and the cane. Regardless, it sends a strong signal, one that I pick up on immediately. I'm going to have to tread lightly.

I gently touch her shoulder, shaking her awake, and introduce myself: "I'm Dr. Thompson. I'm taking over on Maroon 1. I'll be rounding this next one week." I then pull up a chair, sitting down next to the bed. Nothing worse than standing over a patient on rounds; I find it very awkward and somewhat a position of power and authority that might intimidate the patient or family. Not to mention that studies have shown that if you just *sit down*, the patient overestimates the amount of time spent with the doctor by something like 120 percent. Plus, sometimes, honestly, I just get too darn tired.

She takes the sleeping mask off from over her eyes, then slips on tortoiseshell horn-rimmed glasses, but keeps the panda bear hat and blanket in place. She's a petite Asian female, quite attractive, with long black straight hair flowing well past her shoulders, high cheekbones, soft smile—although I can tell by the facial puffiness and the swelling around her eyes that this anasarca is very real. She simply stares back at me for some time, appraising me, taking me in. She then begins to speak in a very soft voice. I simply sit back and listen, keeping my mouth shut so that I can gather more information about her communication style, personality, preferences, and so on.

I can tell right away by her observations and descriptions and questions that she's highly intelligent, articulate, and motivated to learn. She wants to know more than the average patient about their disease or the treatment plan. After hearing, for example, that we are starting a new medication for high blood pressure, it's not just "What is the name of it?" or "What are the side effects?" She asks, "What about the timing of this new medication with the other meds? What target blood pressure are we really aiming for? And if my kidneys are truly shutting down, how will that possibly reduce the effectiveness of the medication, or does it alter the dose or the schedule? Could we instead use that medication 'as needed' if the number goes above a certain range?"

Along a similar vein, she starts asking about blood sugars. "At home, I take long-acting insulin, then eat my meals. Then after a meal, I will take additional short-acting insulin if the glucose is above a certain level."

I respond, "Yes, we call this sliding scale." Instead, the hospital Endocrine team and the nurses are trying to get her to use pre-meal insulin, which is also called carb counting. She's having a hard time with this and describes how her home approach was working so well, although by now, she's so anemic from the progressive renal failure that I think her most recent hemoglobin A1Cs were unreliable. At any rate, she really wants an explanation of why the change. So I say, "There are multiple studies in the medical literature that compare sliding scale to carb counting and find better overall glycemic control as well as fewer adverse events such as low blood sugar. This is a more proactive approach rather than a reactive approach." But also, I mention that this is really more important for the long-term outpatient management of diabetes and less relevant in a hospitalized patient. Still, we try our best to mimic what you should be doing as an outpatient while you are here. She thanks me and tells me she very much appreciates all the information and the insights and especially the medical studies and outcome's data. Amanda asks, "Can you bring me a copy of the journal article you just quoted? I'd like to read it myself." I tell her, yes, I can look it up online and bring her a copy later. "But for now, can we just go back to what I was doing at home?" At which point, I say, "Sure."

Over forty-five minutes have passed, and after I exit the room, I think, *I've got to better budget my time for tomorrow and the coming days.* But thinking back, I'm also impressed. She is quite thoughtful and asking very good, well-informed questions.

I will find out later that she's a data analyst using computer programming to evaluate big data and look for trends and other analysis. This makes perfect sense to me. I see her doing that with her own blood pressure and blood sugar readings, as well as the labs, including the creatinine and hemoglobin. I am so glad I have Epic on my mobile when I am in the room with her because I can quickly access all this data without having to go find the computer and log in.

The next day, I round, again late morning, and when I enter the room this time, the lymphedema specialist is there, helping to place compression wraps around her lower legs to alleviate the swelling. I briefly have a flashback of visiting the lymphedema clinic myself back in June and July, for the axillary web syndrome. At Amanda's bedside, I see a nice young female physical therapist, and I read her name tag as Sara, someone I have never met before now. Still, I mention to her how impressed I am with the lymphedema program here. Once again, I think I am so glad my arm is completely back to normal. Physical therapists are my new favorite healthcare providers—in addition to surgical and medical oncologists. I then say, after snapping out of my reverie, "How are you, Amanda?"

She stares back at me for a few seconds, turns her head slightly to the side, and then states flatly with a sly smile: "I am being mummified."

I just have to laugh. That is a very astute observation. Actually, it sure seems akin to the mummification process of yore, this ongoing lengthy white gauze and gray ACE wrap, round and round, starting at the foot and advancing up both legs. I say, "Well, at this point, Halloween is not that far off. Maybe we can plan a costume for you that kills two birds with one stone!" She laughs too. Ah, success, in my opinion. We've broken through, a little, and I found out that she also has a sense of humor.

Next, the discussion turns toward, again, the blood pressure and blood sugar management. I sit down, and today, her nurse Jackie has accompanied me to the bedside for rounding. This is immensely helpful. I try to make a point of doing this with the nurse every day, but sometimes, we get caught up into other activities and don't get to the bedside at the same time. Jackie has been a nurse on the med-surg ward at the U since I was a *third-*

year medical student. So that's now over twenty years that I have known Jackie. She's instantly recognizable because she has a very large head of hair, a curly dark-brown bouffant; nobody else on the unit has anything quite like it. And now, even with my rare appearances on the wards these days, she always recognizes me. This morning, walking onto 5B, she had said, "Hi, Heather! You have Amanda today? Oh, I know, she can be a difficult patient. But it's so good that she seems to have established rapport with you." So together to the bedside we went.

Amanda comments again on the sliding scale versus carb-counting strategy and how she is grateful that at least for now, I let her go back to her usual home regimen. I had also changed the hydralazine order for blood pressure management to IV PRN instead of oral scheduled, because she is associating some of her symptoms (fatigue, nausea, pounding headache) with the blood pressure fluctuations even though they are more likely to be related to renal failure and volume overload. But still, I'm fine with it. She thanks me for that.

She then launches into a fairly long, detailed explanation, a recounting of events last week. "Whenever I started asking about med changes, it got me into a bit of a battle with the nurses and even that nice young doctor who was rounding last week." Inwardly, I am thinking, *With the rising creatinine, the pending need for dialysis, the progressive volume overload, the ever-changing picture, the moving targets, I am not really overly concerned about either the blood pressure or the blood sugar.* As long as they are not markedly elevated, I would probably agree to whatever the patient wants. *Who cares, we'll get that BP down after the tunneled dialysis catheter is placed and the first few runs pull off tons of volume.* I don't say this, though. I say, "Well, we need to have a treatment plan that you feel comfortable with."

Jackie chimes in and says, "I've been Amanda's nurse for several days now, and she is a very informed, activated patient. I think she knows her own body and what works for her." Amanda nods, then turns to me, and asks, "So why is it that *you two* respond in this way when last week it was nothing but arguments and heated debate?"

I turn to Jackie, looking at her, taking in the streaks of gray in that dark-brown curly bouffant and the laugh lines around her eyes. I also think back to me as a third-year medical student working with her on this very same floor. I turn back to Amanda, and I say, "Honestly? Age." The three of us laugh. I go on to explain that I've been doing this for a while, and I recognize that not every patient is the same. Sometimes there are symptoms or lab abnormalities or blood pressure fluctuations or other phenomena that we can't explain medically, and it's okay to deviate a bit from the standard treatment plan if it just works better for that particular patient sitting in front of us. I also mention, without filling in any details, "I've been a patient myself now, and I am well aware that, on a certain level, there is always a need to have some degree of control over the situation, to have a say in our own medical care." Inwardly, I can recall cutting my blood pressure medication in half without telling anyone; waiting weeks, dragging my feet to start tamoxifen; refusing to wear a compression sleeve as the therapist had recommended during that period of cording on my right arm.

It's been a good morning rounds, and in the coming days, I actually move these late morning rounds to early afternoon so that I can round with not just the bedside nurse but with the nephrologist, Dr. Foley, who is really driving the bus on this case. This works out beautifully—Amanda can ask questions of the two doctors at once; we can respond together, we're all on the same page. Together, leaving the bedside and washing our hands, Dr. Foley comments, "We really should be doing this more often, these joint attending rounds. And not just when a patient is dying and we call a family conference to get multiple teams in the room to weigh in on the prognosis." I couldn't agree more.

So Amanda stays in the hospital, not just for my entire week of rounding but into the next, because of the weekend phenomenon and the delay in getting the dialysis catheter placed. At one point, Amanda mentions transferring all her care to the U. She wants to consider renal transplantation as an option, and given her young age, this seems to make sense. She had at one point scheduled an appointment with Dr. Jill Bowman, my colleague in the PCC who is an outstanding clinician, but she missed it due to the extended hospital stay. So once again, I find I am reaching into my white coat pocket and giving her one of my cards to establish primary care with me as an outpatient. I mention, "Jill's great, but this is another option to see me. It might be a real blessing not to have to tell your story all over again to yet another doctor." She gladly accepts my offer.

That following Monday, I am signing out my team to the oncoming hospitalist, Dr. Paul Kleinschmidt. That's good, I think. He's my age, approaching mid-career, has more clinical experience, and in my opinion, has a bit more relaxed, rational, and very patient-centered approach. In fact, he started a patient-centered communication course that all physicians in our practice are now required to complete. A perfect fit for him to take on Amanda as a complex, challenging, but honestly quite rewarding staff-only patient. He'll put those communication skills to use.

And as I am preparing to sign out, I am acutely aware of how language and words and phrasing can affect the entire transition of care, the handing of the baton. It's even been shown to possibly lead to medical errors. "Framing" is what we call it. When a patient is presented in a particular way that makes the doctor think of only one etiology or one diagnosis or one potential treatment plan, closing the door to other possibilities. I remember back to when I heard the initial wording "difficult patient."

Over the past seven days, I am coming to realize, it's really not Amanda who is difficult. It's the entire medical scenario of a young woman with diabetes for only ten years and hypertension just recently, whose kidneys are now failing and approaching the need for dialysis. It's taking a physically active, working full-time, productive member of society and placing them in a dialysis unit for four hours three days a week. And it's the entire process of evaluation and management leading up to that, including labs, biopsies, scans, vascular access planning, compression wrap treatments, interventions, medications, multiple consultations. Trying to get interventional radiology to place a tunneled dialysis catheter on a Saturday—now *that* is difficult. Not Amanda, really.

So I call Paul, and after running the entire Maroon 1 list, ten in total, I mention, "You also have just one staff-only patient on the Gold 3 list. She's my new favorite patient. I really like her, and I'm also going to follow up in clinic as her primary care doc too, so please, keep me posted on what's been happening even after I leave."

Meet Amanda.

Chapter 17

PROFESSIONAL HELP

We all want to be big stars, but we don't know why,
and we don't know how.
—Counting Crows

E nd of September, I've finished the inpatient week, and I am back in my usual mode at work—clinic five sessions per week and devoting the remaining time to teaching activities, such as preparing to present that board review session in October, gearing up for the six-week course on hematology and gastroenterology in the medical school, and facilitating one workshop on primary care skills for the residents and another on professionalism for the fellows. It's keeping me busy as usual—in particular, the second-year medical school curriculum. As course director, I not only create the six-week calendar, coordinating lectures and small-group case discussions, but I also create learning objectives and frameworks, select course reading materials, and edit practice questions and the final exam. Above and beyond that, recently, I've had both small-group facilitators and large-group lecturers bailing on me at the last minute, so guess who fills in and takes over? Yours truly. Course director, in some ways, could be replaced with the term "glutton for punishment." It sure comes in handy that I am a general internist; I can substitute teach for both Heme and GI topics. And it's a good thing I know the material so well—it's my fourth iteration. Otherwise, I would be in complete panic mode.

While busy is good for me as always, I'm also a bit distracted and certainly up and down in terms of mood. I'm *still waiting* on word from multiple publications relating to the book, including those two chapter excerpts I sent off and, of course, the manuscript itself, which is apparently still sitting on some editor's desk at a local academic press, collecting dust, with a ring of a coffee stain on the title page, a smear of jelly doughnut filling near the corner, for over five months now. Part of me wonders if it has even been read yet by a single editor, staff member, or assistant. I look again at their website, then I see that they have at least a four-step process for all book submissions: first, it must pass the initial editorial screening, then it gets sent out for peer review, then staff evaluation, then a faculty committee, including a member of the board of regents who must vote to approve.

I have a sinking feeling, reading that description. I am envisioning a bunch of academic literary types sitting around a table, wearing black turtlenecks and berets, hoping to review yet another tome on architecture or a textbook on 1960s politics when my quirky memoir lands in their lap. They are probably looking at each other, scratching their heads, saying, "Are jokes about breast cancer even funny? What about all these scripture references? Are we going to offend someone? And the music—do we need John Popper's approval to use his song lyrics? On top of this, she questions some of the design elements of the brand-new Clinics and Surgery Center. Boo! Hiss! We can't have this kind of heretical publication with our name on it!" And here I naively thought that an academic press would be *more* interested in publishing me as a university teaching faculty; perhaps I was wrong. I could have made a big mistake here, wasting months of my life waiting on them. As in:

Monday, September 19, I decide to cold call them instead of sending yet another email. I look up the number for the editor online. I've tried calling this number numerous times before last summer; I was always routed to voicemail, but then couldn't leave a message because the mailbox was full. I assumed this might have something to do with the summer months, so I thought, *I'll try again.* I dial again and I am shocked when his assistant actually picks up the phone and says, "Hello, this is Christopher. How can I help you?"

"Christopher! Hi. Yes. Hello! This is Dr. Heather Thompson. I am on faculty at the medical school. I sent you a book submission back in early June—"

"Yes, I know who you are," he interrupts. "Yes, we need to talk. We've been meaning to get back to you . . . The editor is not in the office today. He should be back tomorrow. Can we call you sometime this week?"

"Oh! Yes. Of course!" I say. "The number that I am calling from now is my cell phone. I also list my office number on the manuscript proposal."

"Great!" he says. "We'll talk more soon!"

I hang up, fingers crossed, immediately emailing Charlie about this conversation.

Then nothing. *Ghosted.* For another four weeks plus, I hear not one word, not via phone nor email nor homing pigeon nor postal owl. Earlier, I had equated the book submission process to pregnancy, then later dating. Now, honestly, it feels as though I am being jilted at the altar. It is causing major feelings of inadequacy. So in addition to work, I simply must find something to fill the weekend time for a while so that I don't get completely down and depressed about the situation. Thank goodness for my two favorite professional sports—the PGA and the NFL. Both are gearing up in a big way this particular September.

Watching the Golf channel and reading Golf magazine, I am getting the sense that there is a lot of hype and energy surrounding the 2016 Ryder Cup to be hosted at our very own Hazeltine National in Chaska starting September 26. Here in the Twin Cities, it's making the local news, local headlines in the paper, getting airtime on the radio stations since we are hosting such a big event. It's creating a buzz and in a very good way.

First of all, the Americans have not won since 2008. They are obviously hungry for a victory. Second, after the big upset, the turn of events in Scotland in 2014, there was literally a task force formed within the US PGA, rethinking the entire Ryder Cup approach. They reinvented the scoring system for choosing players, the pairing of match teammates, the coaching in the form of team captains. Davis Love III, or Trip as he is nicknamed on the tour, is the lead captain this time, and I think he is the perfect fit.

Despite the shortcomings in his personal life, I am still a fan of Tiger Woods. Yet when I see that he is a vice-captain, not a player, I think, *Good. This might be a better role for him. He was a bit too intimidating, not just to the opposing Europeans but to his other fellow teammates as a Ryder Cup player.* Lately, his golf game is completely off. Everyone knows that, but he might make a better captain. Then I go on the Ryder Cup website and see that my favorite veterans and young guns have already made the team—Phil Mickelson, Dustin Johnson, Jordan Spieth, Rickie Fowler, and the Ryder rookie, Patrick Reed. At this point, there is still one final captain's pick that is missing. I pause, I speculate—I really hope it is Bubba Watson. I love Bubba—his passion, emotion, character, even his mullet hair—and watching both Masters wins in 2012 and 2014, he plays amazing golf! But alas, I find out during Sunday Night Football the week prior that it is not Bubba but instead Ryan Moore who made the cut, given his finish at the Tour Championship as a playoff runner up to Rory McIlroy. Never anything less than a team player, Bubba is enthusiastic as ever to support Ryan and is offered a position as a vice-captain instead.

As it turns out, Paul and I had those tickets to the Ryder Cup gifted to us by our school. At first, I was a bit disappointed that it was a practice round and not actual match play, but by all accounts, many say practice rounds are often more fun and more enjoyable than the real deal. Importantly, one can really get up close and watch the players in action, taking pictures or even video of the PGA pros, taking their game to the course. I did this enthusiastically, snapping photos of Phil on the tee box, then recording video of us following him down the fairway. Talk about tiring—trying to keep up with a PGA pro on foot across an eighteen-hole golf course, well, that is a challenge. But I was amazed, honestly, at just watching the entire process of a professional swinging a golf club. Never before had I seen a swing so effortless, so smooth, like butter, with such a soft "ping" at contact but then producing such a powerful projectile, launching a ball over 360 yards on a drive. Also, a fun moment—while walking between holes 16 and 17, crossing a grassy patch of ground, I am almost run over by Dustin Johnson and Jim Furyk in a golf cart. I whip out my phone out of my back pocket and snap a shot that is perfectly in focus of the twosome on that cart, careening left to avoid any collision. Paul sees this and starts laughing. A lady from behind us exclaims, "Well, I guess you have to be prepared for just about anything around here!"

On Friday, September 30, after this very enjoyable outing to the practice round, I am back at work, and I decide to stream live the Ryder Cup for the entire day on my PGA phone app. In between patients, I am glued to the screen. It is unusual, that I am this much into a sporting event, especially to the point of watching while at work. But at the very start, Friday morning, I see the Americans win all four matches. Wow, now that is a statement, really something to consider. I announce to all my colleagues in the PCC at 1:00 p.m., Friday afternoon: "USA is going to win the Ryder Cup this year." Several frown. Jim Langland says, "Aren't the Europeans favored to win?" Alisa Duran agrees. "Doesn't matter," I say, "I saw this team in the practice rounds, and now just watching the first round of foursomes, they are on fire. There is something different, let me tell you. Wanna place a bet?" Nobody bites.

The next day, a Saturday, would have been a great day to tune in to the same format again—four balls followed by foursomes. However, we are taking Sam and three of his buddies to ValleyFair for the day to celebrate his birthday. I am certainly glad I have this Ryder Cup app on my phone. I check it often, standing in line to ride the Renegade Coaster, for example, and now I am getting just a bit nervous. Briefly, the Europeans pull even with the United States—mostly due to the incredible performances from Rory McIlroy and Thomas Pieter. Later in the afternoon, however, the US team would rally, pulled into the lead by Patrick Reed. The loudest roar from the crowd that afternoon came after his hole-out for eagle on number 6. Americans rebound, pulling away to go up 9.5–6.5, entering the final day of the event, which I just know is going to be a nail biter, an amazing finish, no matter what the outcome. And it's the singles round, one-on-one match play, the most competitive and incredibly intense golf in this format.

Sunday: normally, my family attends the second 11:00 a.m. service at our church, especially now with Sam sleeping in until

10:00 a.m., like a typical teenager, every weekend. But today, we have competing priorities, and we rearrange our schedule, planning on attending the 9:00 a.m. service so we can watch the final round of the Ryder Cup on TV. Going to early service, though, proves to be a big mistake as far as the kids are concerned. I can't drag them out of bed and dressed in time to attend. We let them stay at home in their pajamas, watching cartoons, while Paul and I venture out and back. I am feeling a little guilty about that, but I decide we can do a family devotional or something later that evening instead. The Ryder Cup happens only once every two years after all!

And just as predicted, this Sunday of the Ryder Cup is one of the finest and most spirited golf rounds I have seen played recently. The first pairing, Rory McIlroy and Patrick Reed, is one for the record books—the fiery performances, the spectacular shots, both players really energizing the crowds. I simply marvel at Phil Mickelson making ten birdies in his match with Sergio Garcia; equivalent stroke play would have his score at 63. And lo and behold, the last-minute captain's pick—Ryan Moore. He actually clinches the victory by pulling ahead of Lee Westwood in the final moments: on the par 5, number 16 with an eagle; par 3, number 17 with a birdie; and par 4, number 18 with par. The United States dominates, winning back the Ryder Cup 17–11, and on our soil and in my beloved home state of Minnesota!

This again makes headline news nationally, as well as locally. I am driving into work on Monday, and I hear on the radio, "The Americans sweep the Ryder Cup at our very own Hazeltine National here in Chaska." I report to clinic, and I immediately needle Jim Langland: "See! I told you so!" He laughs and says, "You were right!" One of our clinic nurses, Ann, talks about watching the final round on TV with her husband and enjoying it so when the two of them haven't really been into golf much lately. We compare notes about our favorite shots and marvel at the talent of these players. This Ryder Cup high stays with me for days.

Also, during this same month, it's the start of the NFL football season. As it turns out, the Vikings defeat the rival Packers in the very first game played in the beautiful new US Bank stadium, after also winning the season opener at Tennessee. Thanks in part to their amazing defense, they go on to defeat the Carolina Panthers, then the New York Giants and the Texas Titans—and all this despite Teddy Bridgewater suffering a season-ending knee injury resulting in a new QB in the form of Sam Bradford and later another injury taking out Adrian Peterson for the foreseeable future. I dig out my old Vikings jersey and, as usual, watch every single game wearing it but thinking, *If this Sam B. continues to impress, I might just have to purchase a new one.* Number 8 is my new favorite number—as in watching Cam Newton get sacked eight times by that solid Vikings defense. And actually, when I was a child growing up, number 8 *was* my "favorite" number. It's silly, but my birthday is March 8, and I have fond memories of a golden birthday party with everything decorated in gold, including a yellow cake with yellow frosting and candles in the shape of an 8. And of course, just the name Sam B. resonates with me as well— my son. There are two Sams in his class at school. One goes by Samuel, and my firstborn often gets called Sam B.

So I think to myself, *Okay, if the US can come back and win the Ryder Cup in the Twin Cities—and the Minnesota Vikings are incredibly now 5–0, leading our division, as well as the entire NFL—well, maybe, just maybe, there is hope for even little old me striving to publish a book.* Minneapolis Miracles never cease. I'll just keep trying and keep writing and hope for the best.

> But when everybody loves me, I'm going to be
> Just about as happy as I can be.

Chapter 18

CONTINUITY OF CARE

One of the essential qualities of the clinician is interest
in humanity, for the secret of the care of
the patient is caring for the patient.
—Dr. Francis Peabody

A s far as contemplating career choices, I could trace back to a very early stage—perhaps fifth, sixth grade—an interest in medicine. It started out with a love of basic science, including biology; my middle school science teacher, Mr. Randy Johnson, was a particularly positive influence in that regard. Peering through a microscope for the very first time and marveling at the wonders of the paramecium, I had a newfound enthusiasm for observing and exploring the microscopic world. At one point, he gave us an extra credit assignment: scraping the inside of our mouths and staining the slide, looking for squamous epithelial cells, then describing them. At that time, I can recall wondering, What other interesting building blocks are part of the human body? What about the cells that make up muscle, bone, nerve? Mr. Johnson also let me stay after class and help maintain the cultures of Volvox and other algae and protozoa for viewing under the microscope; I was functioning like a lab tech or a lab assistant, which was actually my first "real job" at 3M while in college. Later, my interest in science evolved into a need to apply that science to the human condition, helping people feel better, perhaps even healing them. Unlike many of my colleagues, I did not have any family members in medicine—no doctors, no nurses, not even many with a four-year college degree—so this was all truly new for me.

However, once I was actually in medical school, I had a much more difficult time deciding what exactly I wanted to do with the rest of my life. The first two years of med school were a bit of a blur, a vast amount of material to master in a short period of time. But then, the third and fourth years are comprised of clinical rotations, where finally—finally!—we get to interact with patients and get a taste of what all these years of training have actually been leading up to. The problem was, during that third year, I thoroughly enjoyed almost each and every rotation: general surgery, followed by pediatrics, then OB, internal medicine. At the time, I had thought I could see myself in almost any of these fields. I started to wonder how on earth I was going to choose a career path and commit to a time-consuming and expensive residency application process, when so many of my fellow third years were already set on orthopedics or pediatrics or radiology from the get-go.

At one point, my advisor, Dr. Wes Miller, told me, "First decide on medicine versus surgery."

However, I had a hard time even with that. I say, "I like procedures. I like doing things with my hands. But at the same time, I enjoy the problem-solving, the diagnostic dilemma, the Sherlock Holmes approach to a challenging internal medicine case."

Next, his advice was "Well, then consider a specialty that has elements of both. Perhaps emergency medicine or internal medicine as a hospitalist or a critical-care doc."

That seemed to resonate with me. I went on to rotate at the Hennepin County Medical Center ER, and wow, was that an experience! For a period of time, I became convinced that emergency medicine was the right path for me. But later, I would change my mind and revert back to internal medicine, because of one aspect I would value highly—continuity of care.

I can recall, on my second emergency medicine rotation at Regions Hospital, evaluating an extremely interesting case—a twenty-eight-year-old Hispanic male brought in by a friend for "weakness." This is such a nonspecific symptom, it can almost mean anything; that coupled with a language barrier, and I'm not sure exactly how to proceed or what we will discover, if anything, on the evaluation. It turns out that he has noticeable, demonstrable lower extremity motor weakness, even by a fourth-year medical student's pitiful neuro exam. His labs return with a potassium of 1.7, the lowest level I have ever seen.

Very intrigued by this, I present the case to the attending and excitedly explain, "I think this might be one of the periodic paralysis syndromes. This is definitely something real. I'm looking up what labs to order or how to proceed next."

The ER doc sees the potassium, yawns, says, "Get him on a cardiac monitor, start potassium, and move him up to 8C on Medicine." And so in a matter of minutes, off he goes.

I begin to say, "But wait, don't we get to proceed further? I've been reading... Get *this*, there is a variant of periodic paralysis due to hyperthyroidism and it is more common in young Hispanic males! We should order thyroid function tests!"

But nobody in the ED at this moment in time seems to care. I get the distinct impression, once the decision is made to admit, that's when the thinking stops. I am terribly disappointed, and for days later, I follow this patient via the electronic medical record and discover they do send a TSH and it is undetectable. So it was indeed hyperthyroid periodic paralysis. I saved his name and medical record number, and later I would present the case as a poster at the local American College of Physicians meeting.

So it was back at that point when I realized I have a deep-seated psychological need to follow through, to find out what actually happens to my patients, and that's not very feasible in emergency medicine. To me, there is value in the follow-up and continuity of care that outweighs the higher salary or more "predictable" hours of EM—predictable in that it is shift work. And not just intellectually, as in, knowing the diagnosis, finding out if you were right or wrong; there is even more value in the relationships, the emotional connections, the bonding that occurs when caring for a patient for five, ten, fifteen years—or more. As it turns out, continuity of care has also been shown to positively impact patient outcomes, such as diabetic measures, rates of screening colonoscopy, and so on. Looking back, I am extremely grateful that I did change my mind and chose internal medicine as my career path, even if it was at the very last minute.

In my panel in the Primary Care Clinic, I have two patients that hold my "personal record" for continuity of care: both I have followed since I was an intern in 1998. Yes, that's almost *twenty years* of continuity of care. These two patients are truly on the opposite ends of the age range, medical history, even racial and ethnic backgrounds, and socioeconomic status. But both have taught me so much about continuity.

One is Omar, an African American male with spina bifida and neurogenic bladder complicated by multiple UTIs; I inherited him as a transition from pediatrics to adult medicine at the tender age of sixteen. The first thing I notice, while reviewing the chart, is that this patient practically *lives* in the hospital. Despite his young age, he is admitted about once a month, typically for another UTI, generally requiring IV antibiotics and a two-to-four-day hospital stay. He also tends to get a lot of associated abdominal pain and back pain with a UTI. "Back spasms" is how he describes them. Given his spina bifida, he doesn't have the usual localizing symptoms, such as painful urination, frequency, urgency, and so on. The stress of the UTI will also manifest as autonomic instability—meaning, his blood pressure and pulse will vary widely, and that is another contributing factor in this cycle of frequent admissions. The ER will see the sky-high blood pressure and panic.

And although these are very legitimate reasons to be admitted to the hospital, I also get the sense that Omar also simply enjoys being there. He makes friends with the nurses on the medical ward; he gets to know the unit staff, often sitting in his wheelchair next to the nurse's station on 5A for most of the day, laughing and chatting with the clerks, the RNs, the nursing assistants. There is much in the pediatrics literature about patients with chronic medical conditions that start at a young age, as a child or an adolescent. They tend to have a very "medicalized" existence; their experiences in these formative years are more or less defined by the interactions with the health-care system. As such, their identity exists within these medical interactions, and it is difficult to separate from other sources of personal validation. I think perhaps this is the case with Omar.

But at the very least, having a follow-up with me, the same doctor, for so many years seemed to help with the coordination of care, including discharge follow-up after these very frequent hospital admissions. I answered many a page from our ER (or even outside ERs, such as Abbott) to discuss his case, and I would respond, "Yes, that's a typical presentation for Omar." And I could help guide the treatment plan just a bit. Omar himself began to comment on our long-term relationship: "You've been my doctor for, like, forever!" And when I do my rounds at the hospital, if he happened to be admitted, I would try to stop by. Just seeing a familiar face among the rotating teams would hopefully help. Sometimes, it's the little things, especially for a patient who has been through as much as this.

The other is Gary, seventy-eight years old, a retired police officer and a real gentleman. I had been managing mainly his high blood pressure for many years, but even now approaching eighty, he looks twenty years younger than that. I have seen him through many life challenges—such as being the caregiver for his wife with Alzheimer's dementia and then losing her; later on, the sudden onset of congestive heart failure, leading to the cath lab and eventually bypass surgery; and more recently, slowly losing his vision to macular degeneration. Despite all this, he is extremely fit, exercising two hours every day; his ejection fraction, a measure of cardiac function, fully recovered after bypass. Even more importantly, despite these setbacks, he remains upbeat and positive and so very grateful for his medical care; it is always a pleasure to see him on my schedule.

And wouldn't you know? Gary was the very first patient I saw upon my return to the clinic after breast cancer surgery. That was incredibly meaningful to me, and truly an easy way to start my first afternoon clinic after medical leave; I know his health history and his medication list and can easily recall his recent blood pressure readings—*without even opening the chart*. Typically, I walk into the room and shake his hand, and we get to spend the next twenty minutes out of the thirty-minute appointment chatting about anything and everything: life, health, blood pressure, exercise, the new clinic building, academic medicine, you name it.

Gary's favorite observation of me is this: "I remember when you were a resident and had to leave the room and run everything by your supervising physician, Dr. Susan Diem, then come back in and have her approve the plan."

I laugh and tell him, "Maybe I should still be doing that! Never hurts to get a second opinion, a curbside from a colleague."

But having long standing continuity of care with Gary made me a better doctor in that I was able to connect more with patients, and relate to them on a personal level (even before becoming a patient myself). I also believe continuity played a big role in maintaining his health. From a medical management perspective, I knew which blood pressure meds we had tried and failed over the many years; when he was admitted for bypass surgery, he developed a post-op arrhythmia, and because I had been stopping by for my own informal rounds, I got to discuss in person with his Cardiologist what might be the best management going forward.

Recently, I was able to reexamine the issue of continuity of care in an entirely different fashion. In fall of 2016, I found an email in my inbox, inviting me and two other general internists to a meeting to discuss a new clinical initiative, the Signature Health and Wellness Program. At first, I honestly thought, *Executive physicals? I'm not sure I am interested.* But reading further, I started to consider it; I was willing to hear them out. They were striving for evidence-based, coordinated, patient-centered primary care, and exploring new approaches to preventive health. I thought, *Huh, robust primary care? I've been trying like Sisyphus to push this rock up the hill for years at a subspecialty-driven university. If this type of program takes off, we might be in a position to advance these same innovations or pilot care models in other clinics as well.*

I'm glad I chose to participate because at this initial meeting, at least for me, it's definitely not about executive physicals or taking care of wealthy, high-demand people, or the typical stereotypes surrounding concierge medicine. It's all about continuity of care, coordination of care, and the focus on the patient.

Dr. Bill Conroy, the director of the program, describes the model; he mentions much more focus on diet and exercise, having every patient meet with a nutritionist to review their eating habits and a physical therapist for a fitness assessment. He then goes on to say, "These patients don't want the one-off, the standalone physical. They want someone they can follow up with over time."

I respond, "Well, of course. It's all about the relationships. I've had some patients in my panel for eighteen years. There is simply no substitute for that!"

Then he also mentions, "Patients want a way to access their doctor quickly and easily and not go through a complicated phone triage."

At that point, I laugh out loud; I decide to tell them just a bit of my story, leaving out some of the details but keeping what's important. "I became a patient in our own health system this past year. I came to the U because I wanted the expertise. I chose my doctors for very specific reasons. And I am so glad that I did. I had amazing care. I'm doing great. But I quickly realized that our system is broken. Try getting in touch with a live human being on a Friday afternoon, for example." I explained that because I had my surgeon's cell phone number, I was able to text him and get answers right away, including sending a picture regarding a post-op complication.

I told them, "This has truly changed the way I practice medicine. I have a new appreciation for what patients must endure, the hoops they have to jump through." I mentioned that I've made it a habit to give out my email to all my patients and now even my cell phone number to some. As I was telling this story, other heads in the room were nodding. I could see that everything I discussed was resonating extremely well.

So maybe this new program is a way to put into practice what I have learned myself in the past few months. And secretly, whether M Health realizes it or not, I am thinking, *We need this for* all *patients, not just signature health.* I'm already plotting covert schemes; if I agree to participate, I could possibly leverage my roles in other areas, figure out ways to disseminate this to additional clinics, and maybe even study the outcomes as research and teach it to medical students and residents. Because it's truly the way all of primary care should be practiced; it's just that the system won't pay for it. It takes hiring additional staff to execute this kind of coordinated care, such as previsit planning; taking history from the patient prior to the appointment; ordering the appropriate tests ahead of time so that the doctor can discuss results and give recommendations in real time. Primary care is woefully underfunded in this country, compared to specialty care or procedures, and that is a large part of why executive health programs exist in the first place. Patients who can afford it are willing to pay the extra fee because the United States health-care system simply refuses to do it.

So for now, I will continue my practice in the Primary Care Clinic, fourth floor of the CSC, but float up to the fifth floor several times a month to see a Signature Health patient. I have found both experiences, both clinics, both patient panels extremely rewarding in different ways. I find that I am not really practicing any differently either; I have the same approach and give the same advice. And it's great that continuity of care can exist for both. In the past, I have been on the receiving end of an executive physical report, essentially saying, "Go back to your primary to deal with this." I don't need to do that; I get to hang on to my patients. *I* will be the one to prescribe medication addressing the high blood pressure or low thyroid or the abnormal cholesterol and then arrange follow-up with *me* personally.

I wouldn't want it any other way. And I hope the patients would agree. There is just no substitute for continuity of care.

Chapter 19

Doctors Taking Care of Doctors

Physician, heal yourself.
—Luke 4:23

I am sure it comes as no surprise to the general reader that taking care of a physician as a patient is no easy task. If you search PubMed, there is even a growing body of literature describing the pitfalls of doctor as patient. Much of it involves "VIP" medicine; in other words, as the treating physician, do you tend to alter your care plan or your recommendations based on the fact that the patient is also an MD? Or on the flip side, will the patient be more or less likely to follow your recommendations given their background and training? I found one interesting article, a survey implies that when push comes to shove, many cardiologists don't think the guidelines apply—*to them.* And what about the complexity of the doctor-patient encounter when the patient knows just as much, possibly more than you, about the diagnosis, the treatment options? How does that translate to establishing rapport, discussion of risks and benefits, informed consent, co-creating a plan? Of course, there is no one right answer here. But in November of 2016, in a span of just a few short weeks, I learned that it's challenging; I can describe the highs, the lows, the pitfalls, and the caveats of being in the role of a physician taking care of a doctor. I've been asked to intervene in two separate situations in which a doctor needed urgent medical care. And it caused me to pause and reflect once again on what it has been like for me in that dual role.

Part 1: The Mentor

Dr. Charles Moldow is now a semiretired general internist and former hematologist by training. I've described him in great detail previously as a mentor to me. Charlie has given me career advice; he's read through grant submissions and manuscripts to give me feedback; he's written letters of recommendations for teaching awards, promotion, and so on. Then of course, the relationship changed significantly after both being diagnosed with cancer in the spring of 2016. The deeper conversations and connections about life, death, illness, relationships, healing, the health-care system, and so on—I found them immensely valuable. I truly cherish the bond that we have formed. We often compare notes and experiences on both being cancer survivors, and this camaraderie and mutual support have helped us both cope.

So given this background and context, imagine my concern, fear, angst when—sitting in my office during a visit to campus prior to an Institutional Review Board meeting—Charlie casually mentions, "I've been having night sweats lately."

Alarm bells ring. The first thing I think is, *Good God, Merkel cell carcinoma is back.* In fact, I have just had my own scare of sorts that same week; I've had left-sided low back pain for a couple of days, and I've had to take ibuprofen for it, something that rarely occurs for me. But I've also been exercising more as of late, including spin classes with Dr. Jim Langland, who convinced me to sign up for an indoor triathlon, the University of Minnesota Tri-U-Mah in February. So while it's likely simple musculoskeletal strain, of course, the first thing that pops into my mind is *metastatic breast cancer with a lesion to bone.* After a few days, with some ibuprofen, the back pain has resolved, and everything is back to normal. I think, *Wow, this is how it's going to be for the rest of my life! Every twinge of pain, every new symptom or new concern is going to immediately be related in my mind to cancer. Somehow, I will have to adjust to this, get used to it, and not let anxiety or fear take over.*

But still, given these alarm bells, I ask Charlie more about his symptoms; he thinks it might be a side effect from one of his medications. He's feeling well otherwise, still exercising, not losing weight, no fevers. And with a fairly recent negative PET CT, he's inclined to simply watch it. I am somewhat ill at ease, but then again, I can definitely understand that perspective—to want to minimize the number of unnecessary tests or other workup.

Then, November 2, 2016, late Wednesday afternoon, I receive an email:

> Subject: me
> Text:
> i am unwell
> night sweats (mild)
> fatigue—I could fall asleep standing upright at 3:00 in the afternoon
> migratory arthralgias
> thoracic back pain
> ??ankle edema?? Scheduled to see Cardiology early Dec but these sx are milder yet similar to my bout of bacterial endocarditis 10 years ago. Will check temps. Do you think you can squeeze me in on Friday?? I can come early, wait patiently for your wise counsel.
> Appreciate your thoughts.

I read through this, once then twice, my concern and fear level rising once again. Just the line "i am unwell" bothers me immensely. Charlie tends to minimize his symptoms; I think most MDs tend to do that.

I quickly reply back: "OK I would like to see you tomorrow, anytime before noon, in the PCC. I would not wait until Friday. Will this work? Heather."

His response: "Temp 100.4 today you say jump, i'll be there."

I am reading through these emails again after I leave work and before heading to our usual Wednesday evening programs at our church. On the way, driving there, I am troubled and distracted and contemplating what to do and whom I can call or talk to about his situation. We should certainly evaluate for endocarditis; I've had many patients admitted to my inpatient service with the same situation. But then again, his oncologist will certainly want to know about this. Could it be related to Merkel cell carcinoma? Or the post-op complication that he once had, a seroma? Could that be harboring infection? In my mind, these are all still possibilities. At this point, I am also just a tad frustrated that Charlie's oncologist is someone outside the University of Minnesota, not sitting in the clinic two floors down from me, where I can quickly consult with them and come up with a plan. *I told him not to go outside the U.* I guess I could always call Todd Tuttle, who was also his surgeon.

The next morning, Charlie is promptly checked in at 8:00 a.m.; I am there early as well, and I alert the residents that I will need to see one of my own patients in between staffing their patients. I knock and walk into the room, and he is sitting in a chair, reading the paper, looking very dapper and put together; Gay, his wife, has come along and is also sitting in the chair next to him, nose in a book, as always. We have a long discussion verifying the timeline, the symptoms, and so on. We all tend to agree. This sounds very suspicious for subacute bacterial endocarditis, especially in light of his biomechanical aortic valve, which was replaced in 2007 due to the very same illness. Labs I ordered ahead of time also point in this direction—in particular, the elevated inflammatory markers. Blood cultures were sent, as well, but they need time to declare if positive or negative. I also go ahead and enter an order for an echo, which is scheduled for later that day.

All the while, I am thinking to myself, *Bacterial endocarditis is not typically managed as an outpatient.* There are potentially very serious complications: the burden of infection and multi-organ dysfunction, mechanical obstruction of the valve due to vegetations, heart block if the infection erodes into the conduction system of the heart, or a stroke if a vegetation leaves the valve and travels north to the brain.

I mention this to Charlie. I say, "We really should admit you to the hospital, get serial blood cultures, start IV antibiotics while we wait for results."

"No," he says, "I really don't think that's necessary. This has been going on for weeks. We will know very soon what the echo shows and whether or not the cultures are positive. I can manage. I can go home, and I will come back for a second and third set of blood cultures this evening and again tomorrow morning."

At this point, I have a scenario flash into my mind. We host a weekly conference in the Department of Medicine, Morbidity, and Mortality. As the name implies, it is often used to discuss a patient case where there was an unusual or rare diagnosis, a delay in diagnosis, or a complication, system error, or something else that led to a bad outcome. It's also used for teaching and learning and to prevent similar errors from happening again. The chief resident will select the case, prepare the presentation, and ask questions of audience members; MDs will then comment on the differential diagnosis, workup, or the treatment plan.

I envision the following exchange:

CHIEF RESIDENT: Dr. Heather Thompson from General Internal Medicine, in light of this patient's low-grade fevers and other symptoms strongly suggestive of bacterial endocarditis, can you comment on the rationale of pursuing an outpatient workup?

DR. HEATHER THOMPSON: Well, the patient demanded it.

CHIEF RESIDENT: But isn't the clinical decision-making being influenced by the fact that the patient is also an MD?

DR. HEATHER THOMPSON: Not only that, but he's been my mentor. He's like a father to me, and the prospect of losing him is now clouding my judgment as well!

[Audible gasp from the audience]

Having this in mind, I just have to mention again to Charlie: "We really should admit you to the hospital. When I was last on service, we kept our patients with right-sided endocarditis in the hospital for *weeks*, just to get IV antibiotics without getting sent home with a PICC line to potentially inject with illicit drugs."

He simply laughs and says, "I will stay in touch. I promise to come back late afternoon, and believe me, I won't be injecting IV drugs anytime soon."

I get the feeling he's definitely not going to budge on the admission question.

We conclude the visit, but I don't know exactly what to say. "Call me if you get septic"? Later that evening, I pull up his results in Epic, but the cultures are still pending. The next morning, I am driving into the hospital at 7:30 a.m., and after I park in the ramp, I pull up Epic again on my phone. I see that the first set of blood cultures, drawn at 10:00 a.m. the day before, are turning positive, with a result notification around 6:30 a.m. In a panic, I directly dial Charlie's mobile; he usually avoids talking on the phone, but this time, he picks up right away.

"I already know. I am on my way."

What? I ask him, "How did you know this result before I even did?"

"Dr. Becky Markowitz, the on-call doc—she was paged, and she called me."

Well, I say, "At least this shows our backup system actually works." That encourages me, although I wish they have paged me first. I mention, "I'm teaching a workshop this morning. Then I will come and see you in the hospital later today."

As I exit my vehicle in the parking ramp. I think, *Darn, I just knew this would be the case.* I should have pushed harder to admit him yesterday to the hospital. At least he would have had been monitored, including blood pressure and heart rate and so on. The echo from yesterday didn't show any vegetations, but it did show some stenosis of the biomechanical valve and signs of mild heart failure and fluid overload.

"You could have benefitted from a bit of IV diuretic, especially in light of the ankle edema. I am now kicking myself!" I say into the phone to Charlie.

"I am just fine. There is nothing they would have done in the hospital that we couldn't do at home!" (Other than potentially CPR?)

We talk for a bit more, and after I say goodbye and hang up, I think, *Wow. This is not good. Even if it's nothing related to a recurrence of cancer, it is still very much another setback.* Best-case scenario: weeks of IV antibiotics, potentially at home but still another hassle. Worst-case scenario: the valve will need to be replaced. I'm just feeling for Charlie and his family having to deal last summer with Merkel cell carcinoma, surgery, followed by radiation; and now months later, we are talking about a new problem, more days in the hospital, more follow-ups, tests, and management decisions.

After texting back and forth, Todd Tuttle sends me one additional, very helpful piece of information: Charlie's outside oncologist's email address. I then emailed this doctor on November 2, describing Charlie's symptoms and outlining the workup that I have initiated. On November 11, he replies to it, suggesting an immediate PET CT. There is a saying that relates to medicine: you go to a barber, you get a haircut. Call an oncologist, and you will get a PET CT.

At this point, I think, *Thanks. It's something for future reference, but right now, we have bigger fish to fry.*

Charlie is admitted and started on appropriate antibiotics for bacterial endocarditis. But in typical MD fashion, he is otherwise feeling fine and trying to expedite ways for him to be discharged to home ASAP with a PICC line. This almost worked, until two days after discharge, when his blood cultures yet again turn positive—and these are the sets drawn *after* the PICC line was placed.

This time, it is me who is paged with the result; I call Charlie and say, firmly, "Pack your very best underwear. You are going back to the hospital." He reluctantly agrees. I think he senses I'm not messing around this time.

Eventually, he clears the bacteremia, and although the valve appears to be approaching moderate stenosis, due to his lack of other symptoms and very good exercise tolerance, no further intervention is done. To this day, Charlie is the one and only patient I've ever worked up for endocarditis as an outpatient. Hmm, maybe I can write up another case report?

Part 2: The Bioethicist

Shortly after this episode, mid-November of 2016, a request is sent out from our hospitalist director, Mike Rhodes, needing emergency coverage on a maroon team. I volunteer to pick up a Saturday, Sunday, and Monday since I don't have clinic patients to reschedule. I am rounding at the hospital when I hear about one of our own staff physicians being admitted for acute pancreatitis and the team is somewhat mystified because the exact etiology is not clear; I didn't get any further details.

But imagine my surprise when I get this email from my colleague Dr. John Song: "Hello, Heather. I am the person whom you volunteered to cover. Many thanks. What I am writing about is that my medical history just became a whole lot more complicated. Would you be willing to take me on as a new patient when I am discharged from the hospital?"

It turns out that John has been diagnosed with pancreatic cancer—a terrible disease, usually very aggressive, often doesn't respond well to surgery or chemotherapy. The entire division of General Internal Medicine is in shock, so very dismayed to hear this news, including me. And then I put two and two together, sadly realizing that John is whom the other team has been talking about on morning rounds. This sits with me for days after, bringing about a heaviness in my heart.

But I reply to his email, "Of course!" And since I am rounding myself and I know he is admitted to our own university hospital, I can stop by in person and discuss further. Later in the day, around 5:00 p.m. on a Saturday, I do just that.

I knock on the door as I enter, then look for the foam canister to sanitize my hands. It's my standard routine, yet in this situation, I have such a nonstandard patient. John is sitting up in his hospital bed, laptop in front of him, books and journals spread about the bed and on the table next to it. He looks absolutely no different than when I saw him at Grand Rounds a month ago or when we crossed paths rounding on the inpatient service last summer.

He says, "Heather! Thanks for stopping by! I really appreciate it!"

I find an empty visitor chair in the corner and pull it up closer to his bed and sit. He begins by filling me in on the technical details, including the early presentation of pancreatitis with abdominal pain and an elevated lipase, then the imaging that was somewhat suspicious, which led to ERCP and EUS with biopsy, and now this—a confirmation of pancreatic cancer.

I don't really know how to respond or what to say or even how to begin, and so I revert back to what my doctors asked of me in the early days: "So how are *you* doing?"

He goes on to describe the support that he has from family, friends, colleagues, and also his faith; the pastor at his church has been by to see him multiple times. John also enjoys regular exercise, including running and biking, and has been doing it up until the very day of admission. I tell him, "This is all quite important. We know that functional status improves outcomes, and that mental health impacts physical health."

The discussion then turns toward the treatment plan. He asks me, "Do you think I should seek a second opinion? What do you know about oncology at the U?"

I just have to laugh inwardly; I'm thinking, *Quite a lot*. I mention, "Some of the most outstanding oncologists are here at the university. The best people here would be Dr. Ed Greeno and Dr. Eric Jensen for management of this disease."

We discuss briefly the surgical approach, laparoscopic versus standard Whipple for removal of the tumor. I then have yet another moment where I consider: *Should I share with John that I am a cancer survivor too? Or will that seem irrelevant, just extraneous information with no immediate application to his situation?*

But I also know that John has written extensively about medical ethics; he's published many papers and book chapters regarding ethical issues, he's been recruited for speaking engagements. Thinking about his more public presence in that regard, I decide to open up and say, "I hope this is not TMI, but I became a cancer survivor myself in the past six months. I chose to seek care at the university, suppressing any notion of privacy and swallowing my pride because I wanted the best doctors on the team. I have never regretted my decision."

He responds, "Really! I had no idea. You look so well!"

I explained to him, "I did have good outcomes, and I was very grateful for that, but it was still quite a journey. And it really changed my approach to patient care."

We continue on with the details of his case; I offer to see him in clinic within one week of discharge, or if it ends up that surgery is recommended, I'll work him in for a pre-op.

He expresses gratitude and then says, "By the way, there is no such thing as TMI."

"What?" I ask.

"I've actually researched this as part of my medical ethics training. Most patients want to know that their doctors have been through an illness or something similar. It helps establish trust and rapport—unless, of course, you are a surgeon."

"Really?" I respond. "Interesting! How does that change the situation?"

He explains, "Apparently, patients view surgery as a procedural field, a technical skill. They don't want to think that their surgeon might have a medical issue that affects them, for example, having low blood sugar while standing for long periods of time in the OR, operating."

Ha. I never thought of it this way. I tend to view the thought process of internal medicine and its problem solving equally challenging when compared to making an incision or removing a diseased organ. Dr. Bryan Warren at Regions used to say to our residents, "We need to view medications the way a surgeon views a scalpel. Care and precision should apply to both."

After a few more minutes chatting with John, I decide I have better get going, and I mention that I will stop by the next day to see how he is feeling.

And when I do, entering his room after finishing morning rounds, I don't see him and for a split second, I think, *John must be somewhere off the floor. He's not here. He might be getting labs or imaging or something else done.* But imagine my surprise when I see him suddenly pop up from behind the patient bed near the window; he's doing *burpees*.

"Heather! Hi! I am so glad to see you. Can you do me a favor? Can you talk to the hospitalist team? They won't discharge me because my lipase is still elevated. But I feel fine! Minimal pain! And I am eating a full liquid diet!" (And doing burpees, I think.)

Huh. I find this very interesting, because our inpatient teams admit many cases of pancreatitis on a daily basis, due to the U being a referral center for advanced endoscopic management under Dr. Marty Freeman. As such, we recognize that the typical management of pancreatitis is based on the patient's symptoms and their ability to tolerate a diet, not necessarily the labs. There are good studies in the literature to back this up. Besides, I reason, in this particular case, John's lipase may be elevated for weeks beyond this event, or it may never return to normal until the tumor is addressed. And I can't help but wonder if the team taking care of John is being unnecessarily cautious because he is also an MD. Back to the doctors taking care of doctors dilemma . . .

Whatever the case may be, I want to do my part to ensure that he has the ability to go home and spend some much-needed time with his family. This is another direct extension of my recent cancer diagnosis; no one knows how much time we have left, so for the love of God, let's try not to spend it in the confines of the hospital. I walk over to the workroom that houses the nonteaching teams, Gold 1 and Gold 2, and speak in person to the hospitalist involved in his care.

Now, when it comes to any discussion or potential disagreements regarding the plan, I have always believed that you can attract more flies with honey than with vinegar. So in a very positive, professional, and hopefully egalitarian manner, I say, "Wow! I just saw John Song this morning. I might be inheriting him as a new patient. He looks great! I am so glad he is feeling better. In fact, when I walked into the room, he was actually doing *burpees!*" We both laugh. But I also tell the hospitalist, "Even though he looks well, I know the situation is very serious. I am happy to help coordinate any follow-up on discharge, so that he gets the necessary appointments with surgery, oncology, and so on. If he's tolerating a diet, he could maybe even go home today, Sunday, and I can have my nurse call him tomorrow."

We share a few more observations about John's situation, including the elevated lipase; I offer my opinion that this test may never normalize and it's probably more important to consider the clinical picture. After that, I leave to go back to my office and finish progress notes.

Imagine my relief when the next morning, I look up my patient list in Epic but also click over to the Gold team list—and John's name is no longer on it. I am so very grateful that he was able to be discharged home and recover in his own surroundings. As it turns out, John decides to seek care outside the university, at least initially, and I haven't needed to add him to my schedule after all. But we've still kept in touch, via email, and also a CaringBridge website. Looking back, I am glad that I was able to help out in some small way, perhaps expediting his discharge that late November weekend. It probably reassured the hospitalist taking care of John that I had some connections we could utilize to expedite the outpatient plan, easing potential anxiety about sending him home. Because I now recognize that it can be even more stressful taking care of a physician, compared to the norm, for so many different reasons.

Later, I think back to my own situation. I won't have an appointment with Dr. Anne Blaes until March, four months from now. But these two encounters have reinforced the fact that really, truly, we should do our best to follow evidence-based guidelines, no matter what the situation or how well versed the patient is regarding medicine or the health-care system. Hopefully, I can learn from this experience, and take my own medical training out of the equation when discussing the treatment plans with her.

At this moment, not only was I honored to take care of these two doctors and esteemed colleagues, albeit briefly, but I am also grateful for the lessons learned and the powerful reminders of principles I can apply to my day-to-day clinical practice. Or even my own follow-up, for that matter.

Sure not easy caring for a doctor as a patient . . .

Chapter 20

MY LOVE-HATE
RELATIONSHIP WITH
TECHNOLOGY

Technology is unlocking the innate compassion
we have for our fellow human beings.
—Bill Gates

S hortly after the New Year--January 1ˢᵗ 2017--I heard of
several friends making resolutions regarding technology.
Two of them were giving up Facebook, others were going
on a tech fast, one resolved to take one day off a week (Sunday) as
a break from any and all screen time.

Now, I am not a millennial; I did not grow up clutching a
smartphone. I too, at times, view technology as a double edged
sword, wanting to take a break from it. But interestingly, I also
found I was much more willing to embrace technology after
becoming a patient. I find myself wondering why.

It might have all started with presenting at the academic
meeting in Baltimore, Medbiquitous, about leveraging technology
to improve medical education and patient care. At the time, I was
only two weeks out from surgery, and having so many interactions
with the health-care system myself in the month prior, I couldn't
help but reflect on how better technology could have assisted *me*
and hopefully others by improving the delivery of care, such as

patients having full access to test results and other information in their charts, or easier ways to communicate with their care team.

To this day, I find calling a clinic and playing phone tag incredibly frustrating, and apparently, I am not alone. I just saw a female pediatric emergency medicine doc in clinic. She's been my patient for years. She needed to have shoulder surgery last summer, and when I reviewed the ortho post-op note prior to her appointment with me, I laughed out loud when I read: "The patient is doing well and reports no problems other than difficulty with the call center."

I also notice, when trying to call a patient myself, that it is next to impossible to dial someone's home phone or cell phone and actually have them pick up. There is a reason text messaging is so popular, to the point of carriers providing a voicemail-to-text option. Who listens to voicemail anymore? *Nobody.* And yet, here we are relying on the same archaic modes of communication in the very high-tech, fast-moving, high-risk field of health care. I start to wonder why all our modes of communication haven't reverted to text. In fact, it is sad that my dentist, my hairstylist, and my skin care spa are all way ahead of the curve. They don't call or leave voicemail; they text me appointment reminders and other helpful information.

This leads to an amusing story. Fast forward to end of March; I'm having lunch again with Todd Tuttle, and I mention to him, "It's one year ago this week that I had the abnormal mammogram, then met you in the office, that very first appointment."

He marvels, "Wow! A year went by already! How do you remember these dates?"

And I respond, "I just can't help it. They are embroiled on my brain."

But also I had wanted to meet and ask for his opinion on a potential job opportunity, this new program at M Health, Signature Health and Wellness. I explain they are looking for a somewhat seasoned, midcareer female general internist well connected at the U; and I joking say, being sixteen years on faculty now, darn, I guess that does include me. We chat a bit about that for a few minutes and once again commiserate about the "new" building, still fairly new to us anyway—the CSC in general, including the ambulatory surgery suites—and how that is going. We share a laugh about the new player piano recently installed in the lobby, wondering what's next. A champagne fountain? Circulating trays of hors d'oeuvres?

And while we are sitting at the restaurant, on the table, my cell phone buzzes; it's a patient I have texted, the 4:40 p.m. appointment for later this afternoon. I'm concerned enough about his symptoms of abdominal pain to ask him to come a bit earlier, so that I can order some labs and imaging, and not so late in the day.

The patient responds, "Yes, I can be there at 3:00 p.m."

I send a quick reply, and I tell Todd, "There are a few patients lately that I've given my cell phone number to. I allow them to text me. It's just so much easier."

He smiles and goes on to say, "There was once this patient I saw in the office, and I thought it was okay to give her my cell phone number; but then, after that, she kept texting me with multiple questions when I was in Chicago, then China. On and on it went. She even sent me pictures."

"Really!" I say. "How did you handle it? Was it over the top? I haven't had that happen to me as of yet, anyway." Then I look over at him, and he has a big grin on his face. Suddenly, I turn beet red. *He's talking about me.*

He laughs out loud and says, "I am only teasing you! I'm joking!" I cover my face with my hands. I am blushing so much. Again he says, "It was fine, totally fine!" Now we are both laughing.

You got me. I completely fell for that one—hook, line, and sinker.

But honestly, thinking back, in all seriousness, that was another turning point for me—having Todd's contact information. His cell phone number was so helpful, especially later on. I had sent a digital photo, that picture of my arm, trying to figure out what on earth was happening with a potential post op complication. I just recently asked two of my patients, on separate occasions, to do exactly the same thing: "Please send me a picture." One was regarding a rash on the legs, the other mouth ulcers appearing on the palate. I just needed to get a visual of them, and the text with photo was immensely helpful. There are also certain things you can diagnose by just looking at them, such as shingles. And apparently, axillary web syndrome.

Also, consider the Epic app for smartphones and tablet devices. It truly does save time for my resident team on rounds to be able to quickly glance through the labs, vital signs, medications. Going over to a desktop or bedside computer and logging in repeatedly just takes too much time. Improving the efficiency of rounds led to a myriad of benefits; it expedited orders and consults, moving forward the plan of care for our patients. It reduced burnout and improved morale for the team. And in clinic, Big Epic has gone down for almost an entire day, a total of three times since implementation. It throws the system into a complete state of chaos. But luckily, during this down time, I realized, *Hey, the Epic App on my phone is still working!* I could still see patients and view their charts, even refill medications on this app, but I couldn't enter new orders, such as labs. Still, it was a lifesaver on those occasions.

But if we think our clinic is behind the times in technology, don't get me started on the hospital system equivalent—pagers. The god-awful paging system. I find it interesting that the only people who carry pagers these days are doctors and drug dealers! They are truly dinosaurs in the jungle of technology. Text messaging and the ability to respond quickly via text is infinitely more efficient than getting a page, finding a phone, calling back that number, being put on hold while they find the person that paged you, and having no idea what it's about. And if you multiply that by the sheer number of pages to the interns on our team, one can understand why they average twelve-hour days in the hospital and can't get anything done. An in-hospital phone system with secure text messaging would improve communication and save time. Why this hasn't been done yet is beyond me.

On the other hand, I do wonder from time to time, *Is this use of technology over the top? How will it affect my work life boundaries?* Because with Epic on my phone, I can access work anytime, anywhere—and is that a good thing?

One evening, as I sat at my kitchen table, enjoying a glass of wine, around 9:00 p.m., looking at my tablet, scrolling through social media then email, I see an email message pop up sent from my patient. It's about her recent discharge from the hospital.

I read through it, and I think, *Oh well, it's still helpful to get this information, and I don't necessarily need to respond to it right now this very instant. Everything seems fine. I'll reply in the morning.*

Rarely, less than half a dozen times, a few of my patients have sent me very lengthy emails describing a myriad of symptoms and concerns. This is probably not appropriate; this sort of thing really needs to be evaluated in person. How did I handle it? I sent a very short, one line reply: "I'm sorry you are not feeling well. Let's discuss next time you are in clinic." And that was all that was needed. The brief reply got the message across without creating unnecessary angst, and we should encourage the patient to utilize the correct avenues of care going forward.

More and more, I start to realize that the benefits of technology probably outweigh any downside, but just like anything else, we should encouraged "everything in moderation." I need to enforce some boundaries, just as I try (with varying degrees of success) to limit screen time for my kids. Being mindful about it, planning ahead can help; there are certain times of the day, such as early morning over coffee, when spending half an hour cosigning resident notes from the day before all at once is just more efficient than waiting for them to be completed at the end of the afternoon the day prior. Or when I leave at 6:00 p.m. with an important test result still pending; I'd rather check the Epic app from a restaurant or the local coffee shop and still get to enjoy a bit of a social life rather than wait around in the clinic or log in from my home computer in the basement. But I can see that setting limits will become important, to avoid feeling constantly in "work mode."

The other technology I finally embraced in the summer of 2016 for the very first time was social media. The main impetus was a family road trip to visit the Buum relatives in South Dakota, and since we only get back there once or twice a year with the kids, most were shocked to see how much Sam and Lydia had grown. Many of them chastised me for not posting pics as most families do to keep everyone connected. I used to think that social media would be a waste of time, a real time sink, but after I created my account, I found that keeping in touch with friends and family was just that much easier. I believe my cancer diagnosis actually played a big role in this, too. Not knowing exactly what the future may hold, I felt the need to keep making connections to others around me and deepening the ones that were there and held meaning. Sharing family photos on Facebook reinforced that feeling of connectedness even across the miles. And getting back into writing led me to believe that there is definitely power in sharing one's story, opening up to others; social media is yet another way to accomplish this. Recently, I was even asked to join a Facebook group made up of physician moms who are also cancer survivors. I read through their stories and posts with intense interest; I posed questions and observations to the group and note the responses are immensely helpful. The support and camaraderie is very evident, even though most of us have never met in person.

So 2016 was a turning point for me in terms of technology. Thinking back to the Baltimore trip, I actually took my first selfie there in May of 2016; maybe that *truly was* the turning point! I am standing on a dock in Fell's Point, and my colleague Mark Hilliard is behind me. The entire picture is a bit off center, and I don't even have a smile on my face, but rather a blank stare. It's not very flattering, to say the least. Fast forward to now, and my kids have been teasing me as of late for the sheer number of selfies I have on my phone, taken on both academic and family trips—me smiling in front of the Lincoln Memorial in DC, embracing the Polar Bear at the Coca-Cola Museum in Atlanta, beaming behind sunglasses from the observation deck at Mount Rushmore, poised to hit a golf ball on vacation in Arizona, even my most famous selfie of all: sitting next to Lydia in a roller coaster car, on the uphill climb for the first big drop on the High Roller at ValleyFair. This garnered me an instant chastisement over the ride's loudspeaker: "Put *away* the phone!" but the end result, the photo of us on that coaster, big grins, hair flying in the wind, sun shine reflecting in our sunglasses—well, worth it in the end, in my opinion. Simply priceless.

Huh. Maybe I *do* have some millennial in me, after all.

Chapter 21

A TALE OF TWO OVERS

Well there's a dark and a troubled side of life.
There's a bright and a sunny side too.
—The Carter Family

As I continue my creative writing endeavors, submitting a few essays to academic journals and also working on the book, my family proves to be very helpful. Sam and Lydia read entire chapters, giving me feedback for improvement; Paul gives suggestions for book titles and also articles, and shares opinions on cover art. It's like I have my own mini editorial staff at the Buum house.

One day, Sam was reading along and made this astute observation: "You talk about everything *good* that happened since the cancer diagnosis, but nothing *bad*. People might think you are editing out parts of the story or only telling one side of it."

Wow, I thought at the time, that's pretty profound, *a keen observation for a thirteen-year-old kid.*

I did point out that I describe the fear and anxiety surrounding the early days of the cancer diagnosis and how that tends to rear its ugly head around certain times. But his comment still gave me pause. I contemplated this for a while. Because now, it's almost a year later, and I think: What are the downsides of going through all this? What makes up the low points along my cancer journey after the early days of surgery, medication, physical therapy--

other than the obvious stress of follow-up or some of the physical changes after starting tamoxifen? I don't think my set of tweezers has seen this much use in decades. I thought taming my brow was a challenge; now it's also the chin.

Well, I thought of two "overs"—over identification and overscheduling.

For the most part, this newfound connection with my patients seems to be a good thing; I'm enjoying my work all the more, and my patient satisfaction scores in the clinic actually went up. I received many positive written comments and complimentary feedback in that regard. On the other hand, I must admit, after everything I went through, I can *over identify* with some patients as well. At times, it has taken an emotional toll. Or it's even possible that once in a great while, it may have pushed me to pursue more diagnostic testing than usual.

As an example, there was a young woman with four children admitted to my service a few months back for fevers and enlarged lymph nodes. I was convinced she had lymphoma, which was definitely on the differential; however, her bone marrow biopsy and lymph node biopsy were not supportive of this. The diagnosis was truly evading us, and when I first took over the team, rheumatology wanted to start high-dose steroids for potential treatment of retroperitoneal fibrosis. I was concerned about doing that, probably overly so, realizing that starting steroids could cloud the picture, might obscure the diagnosis of lymphoma that we were still contemplating. Instead, I arranged a liver biopsy given mildly abnormal LFTs and considered going after yet another enlarged lymph node. At the end of the day, everything turned out negative, and by the end of my week on service, she was started on steroids, with rapid improvement in symptoms; the ultimate diagnosis was *retroperitoneal fibrosis*. Was it possible that I was overly concerned, irrationally fearful of missing a cancer diagnosis?

I also had a moment recently when I inherited a new patient; she came to establish primary care with me. She's a forty-eight-year-old woman who, years ago, underwent a bilateral mastectomy and oophorectomy due to the presence of the BRCA mutation. Recently, she developed some upper back pain and was found to have metastatic breast cancer in a vertebral body. I thought, *Really? She went through all this surgery for naught? What a terrible outcome.* And of course, I can't help but think, *This could happen to me.* I've encountered other patients even BRCA negative with my exact stage and treatment who still develop a recurrence years later.

Another patient scenario comes to mind: a forty-five-year-old woman with only a history of intermittent asthma comes in with fatigue, shortness of breath, and a hemoglobin of 5.4. She's labeled initially as a GI bleed, because she had some sort of stomach bug, an acute diarrheal illness in the past three weeks. But upon further history, there was no blood in the stool nor any dark tarry quality to it; and to drop one's hemoglobin *that low*, there should really be more signs. I get concerned when I see the differential of the white blood cell count is also slightly off, the absolute monocytosis; and next the peripheral smear is showing rare circulating blasts. I fear that this could represent a hematologic malignancy. I am also extremely worried that the lab cannot run any routine tests because each specimen is "unable to assay due to interfering substance." There are blood cancers that can produce abnormal proteins.

Because of my concerns, I call for a hematology consult and also transfusion medicine, assuming if this is what I think it is—a possible hyperviscosity syndrome—she may need plasma exchange to remove the abnormal proteins. After pushing a little bit over several days and describing some concerning symptoms (bleeding gums, right knee pain, subtle neurologic changes such as left-hand tingling and word finding difficulties), they finally pursue more labs and eventually a bone marrow biopsy, which confirms the diagnosis of Waldenstrom's macroglobulinemia. This is a condition of high circulating immunoglobulin levels, IgM—in her case, secondary to a lymphoplasmacytic lymphoma.

Now, the academic internist in me is elated and wants to give everyone a high five. This is a rare disease, an unusual diagnosis; I have seen only one in my sixteen years of practice. The resident on the team wants to write this up as a case report, which is a great idea. However, I am simply plagued by the fact, for days afterward, that this is not likely to be a very good prognosis. I read through the doctor's notes, even after rotating off service, and I find that she has only a 30 percent chance of response to chemotherapy. I find myself wondering if she would qualify for a stem cell transplant; she's otherwise so young and healthy. But in the meantime, in the days following plasma exchange, she develops multiple complications of the high blood proteins, including a spontaneous retroperitoneal bleed, a small hemorrhagic stroke. I am no longer happy or excited to have made this diagnosis. I can only think of the fact that she is my age exactly and battling cancer, albeit an entirely different sort. This gets me very down; I have a heavy heart, a sad mood, a negative emotional state, for the next several days.

So at the end of the day, I recognize that I must be careful at times to guard my heart and not take too much of this personally. It doesn't do anybody any good, including my patients and their families, to have a physician taking care of them whose emotional burden is taking its toll. I get distracted when this happens. I fear I will miss an important detail regarding their case or even a separate, unrelated patient case, not to mention being present, in the moment, not just for my patients but my family, my friends, and so on.

The other potential negative outcome of this whole cancer ordeal—overscheduling, getting involved in too many things, stretching myself too thin. This is the opposite of the growing emotional attachment I'm feeling toward my friends, family, even my patients, which seems all the more powerful. Rather than pausing and stopping, contemplating, bonding, connecting, and so on, I seem to be flinging myself into a whole host of extracurricular activities as of late. "Why?" one might ask. "What does that have to do with cancer?"

Well, it's hard to describe, but even with favorable outcomes, I have this overarching sense of pressure, a timeline, almost as though a clock is ticking. Nobody knows how much time we have left—including me, now a cancer survivor. I need to keep doing *this* as long I still can, no matter what "this" might be: running, singing in a choir, volunteering at church, participating in Bible study or mom's group, serving on the school board of directors. The list goes on. It even carries over at work; if I'm asked to present at an academic meeting or teach yet another lecture or take on another medical student in clinic, I will enthusiastically agree.

While at first, it all seems great, at one point, I review my Google calendar, and I just have to laugh. I have all these events listed (and most even span the weekend). I have a national meeting on April 19–21, DC; two-poster presentations. Immediately after that is an Oratorio concert week involving a dress rehearsal, two recording sessions, followed by a Friday evening performance. Next is a Liberty golf tournament fundraiser for the first weekend in May. And oh, by the way, another presentation for Best Practices Day, two days prior to the golf event, discussing teaching innovations at the medical school. Soon after, I'll have to travel to Atlanta with my colleague Mark Hilliard to present at AAMC. It's a bit crazy.

I start to realize this overscheduling is taking a toll as well. Mentally, it's tough to keep track of all the details. I completely forget to make reservations for the hotel in DC, and by the time I remember, the hotel is full. So I have to book another location, paying a very steep price as a result. My family is starting to notice time spent away from them. It's getting to be a bit much.

I sit back and pause and contemplate and realize, once in a while, I may need to simply *say no*. I may need to cut back, slow down, unplug, stop doing at least some of this for a short period of time; I fear I might simply get burned out. I contemplate not signing up for the Liberty Golf Tournament but instead contribute money toward it or let my sister-in-law play in my place.

I even look ahead and consider choir and the fact that I may need to sit out of Oratorio for part of the regular season in the coming years. This is mostly due to the kids' activities, including school, sports participation, church—basketball season in particular. Summer chorus will still be very doable. It's a smaller time commitment (four weeks of rehearsal followed by one performance), and it's usually a major choral work that I have sung before, such as Mozart's Requiem. Summer is also so much more relaxed, not nearly as many activities going on. Or I've even thought maybe the choir trip to Italy next summer should be the highlight, the finale, the ending point of my singing career; I'll really go out with a bang.

I even start to consider what my career might look like if I choose not to go up for promotion. Several of my colleagues have declared this position; they are clinically active—seeing patients and teaching—but not writing grants or submitting workshop proposals or getting papers ready for publication. I consider this fact and wonder just how "freeing" that is from a time and pressure and work-life balance perspective. It's the constant low-level distractions, the multitasking, that seems to produce unnecessary stress.

I start to contemplate the idea of taking a sabbatical instead. After receiving an award, a fellowship to transform our second-year curriculum to fit an active learning classroom, I begin to think, *This is great, but how am I going to find the time to do it? What about a semester leave or a sabbatical? That's a thing, right? Not that I wouldn't be working. I'd be in my office every day! But a temporary hiatus from patient care to focus on one project—now that would be amazing.* On the other hand, I worry about leaving my patients behind. Whom would they see in my absence? Then again, I have taken two-, three-month maternity leaves, and most of them stuck with me. Even a three-month sabbatical would be extremely productive.

At this time, I have no easy answers; I'm sure this is typical of a career in academic medicine, wearing too many hats, being pulled in too many directions. Part-time status also carries a lot of appeal; if I had Mondays off, just one day during the week to catch up would make the weekends so much more appealing, I'll have time to truly relax and recharge my batteries as opposed to just running errands.

After surviving cancer, many patients report their outlook on life is a bit different, or they describe a shift in priorities. I think that is what is happening in my case as well. I will have some decisions to make in the near future in terms of work, career trajectory, extracurricular activities, and so on. I just hope that the life lessons learned from cancer can help inform my approach going forward.

And at the very least, I need to always remind myself to avoid the two "overs."

Chapter 22

CANCER-VERSARY

You're shining, I can see you
You're smiling, that's enough
I'm holding on to you
Like a diamond in the rough
—Shawn Colvin

T his is a tale of a trilogy and a ring—but there are no hobbits, elves, or dwarves involved.

At this point, I am approaching the one-year anniversary of being cancer-free, which is April 26, and I am writing three books. Book 1 is complete; it's all about the early days of my cancer diagnosis. It is still sitting at a local publisher, under review for months and months. *God only knows* why it is taking them so long. Of course, I understand that there is a process here; but I honestly fear I might have a recurrence before I hear back from them, and that could completely change the storyline! Or maybe I will die before they make a decision; this actually might have some sort of potential benefit. Are not most authors or artists even more famous after their death? Perhaps then it could be published posthumously and all the proceeds donated to breast cancer research.

Book 2 has a sixty thousand word count, almost complete, mostly about my patients and my teaching; I have even started writing book 3, one that is probably not fit for public consumption. It's more of a journal, a private collection of stories that reflect the intense emotional roller coaster I've experienced and the changes in relationship dynamics that have occurred in the past twelve months. But now—voilà!—it's a trilogy! Every important work, every project, every key concept can be broken down into three or comes in threes: the tripod, the Triple Crown, the trifecta, the Holy Trinity, the triple aim, the triplet in music theory—you name it.

But back to the trilogy and the ring. I have done something in the recent past that is rather unlike me.

Many months ago, I began to think about the fact that my surgery date was the same day as my wedding anniversary, April 26. At the time, back in 2016, I had thought, *How ironic and sad. Cancel those dinner reservations. I might not be able to eat, with potential post-op nausea and vomiting. I'll still be half drugged from the anesthesia, so no celebratory glass of wine.* And the traditional gift for the thirteenth wedding anniversary—lace—even that is bitterly ironic. I would usually think of a lacy bra or a teddy or some type of fancy lingerie in that setting, and on that particular day, I'm going to have a brand-new ten-centimeter incision, a bloody gash on the right side of my chest, coupled with a drain and a dressing. No way I'm tucking all that into some expensive negligee and then ruining it with a serosanguinous stain.

So even back then, when I was extremely anxious and stressed, and a big "celebration" was the furthest thing from my mind, I was still just a little bit miffed. On the other hand, I decided not to change the date, for some odd reason. I guess in part I just wanted to get the surgery scheduled and be done with it, get it over with; but another part of me began to think that maybe this can, and should, start to augment and supplement the wedding anniversary. The date of April 26 would become all the more important, meaningful, and significant to me. It's a new anniversary altogether; it's also the anniversary of being cancer-free. My daughter even coined her new term for it: "cancer-versary." Love it.

And there is a small part of me, just like any woman (if they care to admit it), that wants to be given a very nice gift to commemorate this. I look up the traditional gift for the fourteenth anniversary, and it is ivory. How very boring, in my opinion, unless we want to invest in a Steinway piano; but our Yamaha U1 sounds great and fits perfectly in that corner of the living room, so no, that would be a waste of time and money.

I think, *Maybe bring back lace?* But at this point, I've already stocked my wardrobe with all kinds of new lingerie involving the soft-cup bras with removable pads. I've graduated beyond athletic gear and now have found similar bras in pretty floral patterns, or lace, in many styles, multiple colors—pink, black, red, gray. Wearing them makes me feel feminine again, and after adding the extra pad on the right, looking at my silhouette, either in my underwear or in clothes, perfect symmetry. No one would ever know I had surgery. It's a grand façade! I've even found several teddies and two pretty nightgowns complete with lace trim and a bow that all have the same soft-cup, removable-pad bra inside. What a concept! It's like they were made for a woman post mastectomy without the manufacturer even realizing it.

So I definitely don't need to add anything to my lingerie wardrobe in that regard. And then, later on, as I began to contemplate the upcoming one-year anniversary of being cancer-free, the number one (1.0), all at once, I have an idea pop into my mind.

Years ago, for our ten-year anniversary, Paul suggested upgrading the diamond in my ring, from a 0.6 carat to a 1 carat, but then we didn't for some reason or another. I think honestly, at the time, I was the one dragging my feet. Part of me didn't want to spend the money; it just seemed a bit frivolous. But fast forward to 2017, and I am thinking, *Yes, I want to celebrate this date.* I want to commemorate it but now for an entirely different reason. I start to think, *I am going to ask Paul for that upgrade.* And again, it will symbolize to me not only the marriage but something completely new and different—defeating breast cancer.

So one Saturday afternoon in February, when there is nothing going on and my family is all just lying around the house, watching college basketball, I suddenly say to Paul, "Let's go to Arthur's Jewelers and look for a new diamond." I know we've talked about it before, but still, with this rather spontaneous suggestion, surprisingly, he's game. We hop in the car, drive the six blocks, and at around three in the afternoon, the place is actually quite busy, probably because of upcoming Valentine's Day. We are greeted by a woman named Justine; we are poured two glasses of Chardonnay. I gravitate toward the "diamond bar," where all the loose diamonds are stocked, and I tell Justine I am looking to upgrade my ring to a 1-carat diamond. Nestled in the middle of this extensive diamond bar, on a small black velvet cushion, is one diamond that is exactly 1 carat.

She pulls it out and reads the description; it is off the chart in terms of the cut, color, clarity, all those "things" they measure that are a bit puzzling to me. But when she takes this gem out of the case and places it on a tray and, to compare, lines up several others alongside it, well, it is definitely impressive. It's breathtakingly beautiful, and because of the flash and the brilliance and sparkle, it actually looks much larger than the 1.2 carat sitting next to it. We get to view it held loosely in a prong setting; she holds it up via calipers next to my ring to compare. It's lovely, so intense that tiny flashes of rainbows are gleaming out as it catches the sun. I move around the jewelry store, looking at it in different levels of light, taking in the brilliance and beauty. It really doesn't take much longer, and I think, *This is the one.* Literally, it's 1.0, not 0.9 or 1.1. I'm done. Sold. Justine is very impressed by my quick decision-making, although she seems somewhat puzzled by my absolute insistence on a diamond that is exactly 1 carat.

I then show her my ring, and because it is a bezel setting, which is more rare and unusual (that's why I chose it), she cautions me that this is going to be a bit more complicated than a prong setting. The bezel itself will have to be cut out, then the platinum melted down, then the entire circle bezel recast around the new 1-carat diamond, then reattached to the body of the ring itself, which from the top is shaped somewhat like a bow and from the side looks like a Crown Royal bottle. And oh, by the way, Arthur's will need to keep my ring for six to eight weeks to accomplish all this. I'm very surprised; I've been thinking six to eight *days*. But off it goes, and I mention to Justine, several times, that the ring must be ready by April 26, at the very latest, emphasizing the importance of this date. But in my mind, it is not just because of the wedding anniversary.

So for a period of time, I'm running around without my rings on. Charlie has once teased me about this, asking me if I have made any new friends during this time period. And I don't know how I will react, honestly, when I slip on this new version of my old ring. I am not usually a girl who goes after bling in that sense of the word; that's why this entire scheme is a bit unlike me. I am not exactly sure why I am doing it. At times, it seems almost devious, a bit self-serving in many ways. But then again, I think to myself, *Other people on blogs and websites describe trips to Europe or buying a new sports car or all sorts of ways to approach an anniversary date related to cancer.* And if we stick with my original idea—a variation of the traditional gift, ivory—well, a Steinway costs much more than this "version 1.00," even a used upright. And in retrospect, I really should have done this back in 2013, just to be able to enjoy wearing it a little bit longer.

Also, the diamond symbolizes to many people the beauty that emerges out from under extreme pressure, a triumph over adversity, a flash of brilliance born out of trials and tribulations. This is how it has been for me. It's how I view things as a cancer survivor. Whatever the future may hold—regarding my health, my career, my relationships—I sincerely hope that God will use this experience to shape me, mold me, make me a better person, despite my shortcomings, my faults, my flaws, my inclusions. In a sense, He's creating a diamond in the rough.

And the inner material girl says, *Hey, after all is said and done, it's simply a beautiful ring.* It's still a wonderful gift, a memorable present, a symbolic keepsake for commemorating this next phase of my life. In fact, when I return to Arthur's to pick up the ring, just two days before the actual cancer-versary date, I finally tell Justine the reason we've decided on the upgrade and why exactly one carat is so important to me. She lets out a little gasp, has tears in her eyes; she leaves the floor and returns with two glasses of champagne. I slip on the ring, which looks absolutely stunning to me, truly amazing. The new diamond is the perfect complement to the bezel setting. We both marvel at how beautiful it is, and Justine congratulates me, gives me a hug; I feel as though I am getting married all over again.

Now I have a new and lovelier piece of jewelry to wear on the fourth finger of my left hand. Staring at it, I will contemplate how much everything changed for me that April 26. Every time I see it, I will be reminded that I am a breast cancer survivor, one year out—and hopefully many more, God willing. It will add even more meaning to this ring and its diamond. Very complex, convoluted, but still poignant and significant, nonetheless.

Happy cancer-versary.

Chapter 23

To Sleep, Perchance to Dream

In the middle of the night
I go walking in my sleep
Through the valley of fear
To a river so deep...
—Billy Joel

There is a saying in medicine residency: everything gets worse at night. It is, like many clichés, amazingly accurate. Pain, fever, delirium, hypotension—whatever the patient is experiencing—it is worse at 2:00 a.m., and that is why the cross cover pager goes off constantly, to alert the doctor who is least familiar with the patient that the crap is hitting the proverbial fan. Cross cover was never for the faint of heart; we used to have a mantra of sorts: "Keep 'em alive until six thirty-five." Sign out, of course, is at six thirty. I am glad that in recent years, overnight call with cross cover has largely been replaced by night float. At least the same doctor is monitoring the patients each night, often seven or more nights in a row—terrible for circadian rhythm but better for patient care.

In April 2016, after I was diagnosed with breast cancer, again everything got worse at night: fear, anxiety, even post-op pain. Prior to any treatment, it was the intense stress, the worry, mostly fear of the unknown, waiting for test results, waiting for the plan, lying in bed, staring at the ceiling. When I couldn't sleep, I tried a mental distraction technique, the alphabet list—a favorite of cognitive behavioral therapists. But I also made a list in my mind, which I called the million-dollar questions.

What type of surgery should I have?

Do I opt for reconstruction?

What about contralateral prophylactic mastectomy?

If I keep the left, will I be kicking myself down the road, going through the same thing on the opposite side?

Is this genetic? If so, what about my kids? How can I help them, protect them? What should I even *tell* them (they're age eight and eleven) if testing is positive?

Will I need chemo? Radiation? If so, will I feel like death warmed over, or will I be able to work? To function? I am a mom and a full-time physician. I cannot be taken down by docetaxel and Cytoxan.

Early on, I found that a half tablet of Benadryl or three milligrams of melatonin really did help. But then, when I actually could get some sleep, the dreams . . . Suffice it to say, I had numerous dreams during that time period I will never forget. Months later, I can recall them with a level of detail that usually evades me by around 10:00 a.m. the next morning.

The first cancer dream: I'm going about my work, my life, my activities; but the entire time, I'm holding a baby. This baby is strapped into a carrier, a Baby Bjorn as I used to wear, a true godsend of an invention, a handy way to hold a baby close while still having your arms free, moving about, doing everyday tasks. So even the fact that the infant is strapped into a Baby Bjorn is symbolic—being a mom yet doing everything else at the same time.

But in my dream, I never get to see this baby, he/she is facing out and away from me the entire time; in my view, all I see is that baby is completely dressed in white, head to toe, including a soft white knit cap. I keep looking down upon it, even planting a kiss on top of it.

In the dream, first I'm at work, and I ask one of our clinic nurses to hold my baby while I check something in Epic. She responds, "I have a walk-in patient I need to see." Next, I'm at church; I try to check my baby into the nursery so I can listen to the sermon. The sour-faced woman at the desk responds, "You haven't registered in our system yet. You will need to keep the baby with you in service." At one point, I am at my parent's house; I ask Mom to hold this baby, and she says, "I was just about to get dinner started. My book club is coming over."

So apparently, in my dream, I am asking for help. Will anyone please come and lighten this load, just for a few minutes, and carry my burden, take this off me, even temporarily? The answer essentially is no. And I am fairly certain the baby, all soft and dressed in white, strapped to my chest, represents the tumor I palpated that fateful night.

The other cancer dream I won't forget is the parking ramp assault. In this dream, I am about to leave work for the day; it is late, the sun is setting, and for some reason, earlier, I had to park on the roof of my parking ramp. As I exit the elevator and look for my car, I see the large red SUV sitting in the middle of the row, but the rest of the area is deserted—no vehicles or people to be seen. I walk toward it, clicking the unlock button on my key, hearing a chirp.

Suddenly, out of the shadows, a man starts running at me. He is tall, thin, pale and has short dark hair and very large, oversized, thick-framed glasses—retro style, like a pair of Ray Bans, or Warby Parker frames. I freeze in my tracks as he runs up beside me, trying to grab my purse. But as he's pulling at the black satchel hanging off my left arm, in my right hand, I am still holding my keys.

I make a fist and take a swing at him, keys pointing out, aiming right toward those thick-framed glasses, with a force unlike any other, a strength I don't know I have. In my dream, I can actually feel the anger, the rage bubbling up inside of me. My punch lands square in the middle of his glasses, shattering the frames, breaking the lenses into a million pieces, and the set of keys bursts open at impact, scattering my keys in every direction. The man runs off, and I am standing there alone, purse still in hand, completely dazed at what has just happened.

Then the most interesting part. I get down on my hands and knees and crawl all over, feeling the concrete, looking for my keys. Eventually, with time, I find each and every one of them and wind them back onto my keychain. First, the key fob itself for me to unlock my vehicle. Then, the key to my office that says, "University of Minnesota, Duplication Prohibited." Next, my house key, then the key to Mom and Dad's place. After that, the smaller key that fits Sam's bike lock. Then the tiny key to Lydia's journal that she asked me to hold on to for safekeeping.

This one is fairly obvious; even Freud would have an easy time with it. Take that, cancer! You won't steal anything from me! I will fight you off and put the pieces of my life back together!

Later, even after the return of some good news and favorable test results, insomnia reared its ugly head again: nighttime hot flashes after starting tamoxifen. Gradually, however, I adapt, these symptoms subside, and after a few months, they are almost gone; I am back to sleeping fairly well.

Approaching the one-year follow-up, though, *again* everything gets worse at night. There are too many thoughts racing through my mind, some of it sheer reminiscence. I'm recalling those early appointments, the crazy whirlwind of events, many emotionally charged. They are embroiled on my brain as such. I look at the calendar, passing by milestones, and think, *March 31, mammogram. April 5th, MRI. April 7, oncology appointment. April 26, operation.* I will never forget these new anniversary dates. I keep thinking of my daughter's term for it: "cancer-versary."

Then, just exactly as before, insomnia—too much time staring at the ceiling—leads to more million-dollar questions; these questions are perhaps not quite as "big" as the first time around, but still as numerous.

What type of imaging should I have? Is 3D mammography really almost as good as MRI? How long should I stay on tamoxifen? When is the peak risk of recurrence? Am I ever out of the woods? I haven't had a period in almost a year; am I technically in menopause? Or is this somehow different? What about bone density? I've read about increased risk of a second malignancy; does this affect other screening? I think back to my radiologist, the fifty-three-year-old woman who shared she had metastatic disease at her first colonoscopy.

Million-dollar questions. Then the dreams . . . I start to have bizarre dreams all over again.

First, I dream Dr. Anne Blaes orders a PET CT for reasons unknown given my early stage, and it shows I have metastatic disease everywhere, including malignant ascites. Dr. Todd Tuttle sends me a text, offering to tap it for me. This is followed by a more realistic dream; there is some ill-defined density in the left breast on imaging. I am referred for a biopsy, and I think, *Here we go again. I knew I should have gone with the bilateral approach!*

But that one is followed by a more bizarre dream—about the triathlon, the Tri-U-Mah, which I completed end of February. I am rushing into the locker room to change in between the swimming and cycling portions of the competition. I need to completely disrobe and dry off and get into bike gear; I am looking in a full-length mirror while doing this, surrounded by other women, all in a big hurry to change. However, in the dream, *I still have my right breast.* I see it myself—both—as I look down at my feet while getting undressed and again as I glance toward the mirror and take in my reflection. How very strange.

I've also had dreams about revealing my diagnosis to my colleagues. In one, it is now fall, and I must report to the fifth floor of my clinic building for an employee flu shot clinic. I go upstairs into a big reception hall full of tables, where all the doctors and nurses are getting vaccinated. Everyone from M Health is there; the room is packed. I sit down at a station to receive my shot, and instead of just rolling up my sleeve and exposing the deltoid, I take off my shirt and bra. I am completely undressed from the waist up, thinking, *Gee, everyone is going to see my mastectomy scar.* An RN approaches me and says, "Dr. Thompson, you don't need to take everything off! Just a bare arm is fine!" And I grab my top and cover up again.

Approaching the one-year follow-up, I have a similar dream. An EKG is ordered prior to my appointment; why, I don't know, but I dutifully schedule it. I am rounding when I get a page from the cardiology fellow, Marina, who was once my resident in clinic.

"Dr. Thompson! Hello! I'll be doing your EKG this morning!"

I leave my team, saying, "I'll be back in half an hour."

I go downstairs to the second floor. I am checked into a room; as I start to undress, needing a bare chest to place the EKG leads, I realize, *Uh-oh. Marina is going to see my scar. She will know I am a breast cancer survivor.*

In the dream, I disrobe, but only down to my athletic bra; I am searching around for a gown to cover up, and for some odd reason, I am starting to panic.

At that point, a technician comes in and states, "You'll have to come back another day. Our EKG machine is broken."

I sigh and start to have more of a sense of calm again.

Speaking of calm, I did have one dream during this time period that is rather fuzzy; I couldn't recall nearly as many details. But despite the fuzziness, the vague recollection, the in-and-out-of-focus quality, I held it in my mind the next morning and in the days to follow, because it had such a palpable emotion attached, suffused throughout—a feeling of calm.

In this dream, I'm up at my uncle's fishing resort in Canada. He doesn't own it anymore, and the cabins and the main lodge have been completely redone. But in my mind, it looked exactly the same as when I visited growing up: the dark-green cabins, the surrounding clear blue lake, the tall pine trees. My family is there; we are all in a boat, fishing. With lines out, we are slowly trolling along, water lapping up against the side. The sun is shining; a panorama of sparkling light is playing out behind us on the rippling waves. I am sitting back, one hand on the pole, looking around at the beautiful scenery and the pristine wilderness, taking it all in. None of us say a word in this dream that goes on for quite a while. We simply turn to one another from time to time and smile.

Peace. Calm. Serenity.

I remember waking up from that dream, early morning, feeling so content and thinking, *Ahh, I just want to fall back asleep, continue on with it. I want more of this kind of dream. No more cancer dreams, please.*

Later, I pause and reflect how despite my medical training, or maybe because of it, I will likely continue to experience sleepless nights and strange dreams around certain times—in particular, anniversary dates or anticipating follow-ups. Just as many of my patients who are also cancer survivors do as well, I am sure; I have come to realize it never really ends. Having this common experience instilled in me more empathy and a new appreciation for what we put patients through—in particular, the incredible burden, the weight of the fear of the unknown. And since, as Osler once stated, all medical care is, to some degree, the unknown and is fraught with uncertainty, it is helpful to recognize how that might manifest, including periodic and predictable bouts of insomnia.

At the very least, I can recommend Benadryl or melatonin, or I can teach my patients the alphabet list.

To sleep, perchance to dream . . .

Chapter 24

DOCTOR AS WRITER

Medicine is my lawful wife and literature my mistress;
when I get tired of one, I spend the night with the other.
—Anton Chekhov

E leven months, nine days, five hours, twenty-nine minutes,
eighteen seconds—that is how much time has elapsed
since I was diagnosed with breast cancer. All due credit to
the handy phone app How Long Ago.

I read those numbers on the display, and it seems so abstract.
In some ways, those days have gone by in a blink; it's been almost
a year, yet it feels like just yesterday when I was trying to hold
very still in an MRI scanner to obtain high-quality images and
decide on the next steps. In other ways, I can hardly remember
life before breast cancer; it seems as though it's always been a part
of me—in the past, now, and forever. I am truly grateful to be
on the receiving end of good outcomes; I appreciate my overall
health, trying to take better care of myself through diet, exercise,
and so on.

But still, as time goes by, I often feel the need to pause,
reflect; I also have frequent moments when I simply stop and
marvel at the life lessons cancer has taught me. So many things
to contemplate, and what better way to do this than through
writing? I've come to realize how much I need writing; it has been
incredibly therapeutic, enjoyable, fulfilling. I even start to make

another extensive list in my mind, similar to my million-dollar questions.

I realize I'm becoming a writer as I notice the following things happening to me.

I burn through not one, not two, but three wireless keyboards in less than twelve months. I've never owned a laptop, but my iPad and Google drive has served me very well in this regard, except for the high turnover of that darn keyboard.

I'm looking forward to two weeks off after surgery so that I could keep writing at home and in local coffee shops.

A six-hour delay in an airport seems enticing or spending an extra day at an academic meeting, holed up in a hotel, typing away.

I start to notice bookstores all around me—such as the tiny independent bookstore on Washington Avenue, Daybreak, right down the street from my clinic building; or the small storefront on main street in my hometown of Milaca, Bexter Book & Copy, with the calico cat sleeping in the window.

When I receive a book as a gift or on loan from Mom, I immediately flip it over, looking for the publishing house. I will then open the cover and read with interest the standard Library of Congress description, the publication date—none of which I gave a hoot about before.

At an academic meeting where the theme is work-life balance, I attend every workshop and breakout session devoted to writing and the therapeutic aspects of it, including ways to promote reflective writing in our everyday medical practice.

I change my profile picture on Facebook to one of me, late in the evening, sitting in front of my iPad, earbuds in place, big smile, getting ready to write after my kids are tucked into bed.

I seek out other writers—my colleague's spouse, who writes children's books; my fellow Oratorio Society member, a bass singer, who recently published a book. I meet a colleague for coffee at the Loft Literary Center, and I contemplate joining a writer's group.

I push myself to continue reading, and not just medical journals; my bedside nightstand is stacked with books. I recently finished *A Man Called Ove*, have moved on to *A Gentleman in Moscow*; next *All the Light We Cannot See*, followed by *The Woman in the Window.* Part of the reason I read is because I think it improves my writing. Observing different writing styles, literary tone, voice, and so on—it strengthens and solidifies my own approach.

As far as inspiration for writing, if I experience something moderately significant in my everyday life, I will mull it over in the days to come, replaying it in my mind. Pretty soon, I feel a theme developing, a corresponding narrative forming in my head; then a chapter starts to coalesce. The thoughts swirling around in my mind are almost similar to a developing tornado. The sky begins to darken. Winds are gathering. A wall cloud forms, then a funnel, then *touchdown*. Boom! Chapter 19.

Writing starts to influence my documentation in the EMR. My own charting starts to take on much more descriptive vocabulary: "Ms. West returns from yet another hospitalization, one of many for the conundrum of recurrent GI bleeding on warfarin, the source of which evades the diagnostic capabilities of the most-skilled endoscopists at the university." At least no one can accuse me of using cut and paste, templates, or dot phrases for *that*.

Writing even informs how I instruct medical students to compose a history and physical or a progress note. With my students, I continually emphasize the importance of a true narrative, a "story" tying together the patient's symptoms, potential etiologies, diagnostic and treatment plans. We even discuss "illness scripts," in which a typical presenting pattern will lead toward a specific diagnosis, and these scripts depend on including all the important elements in the story.

Given all the above, I decide to just run with it. I'm a physician by training, but for some reason, becoming a writer and becoming a cancer survivor occurred at exactly the same time; and now the two are inextricably linked somehow.

In fact, with the roller-coaster ride I've described very early on in book 1—the ups, downs, twists, and turns regarding the cancer diagnosis—I found myself later thinking, *Ha, that is nothing compared to trying to get a book published*, especially a memoir, because as rejection letters pile up, it starts to feel personal, as though it's *me* that's being rejected, not the book; it certainly takes its toll. Those prompt email replies—abrupt, almost rude from several publishers, stating they wouldn't even consider a book proposal from a first-time author without an agent—they are discouraging, to say the least—truly undermining my confidence.

Later, I hear a tentative yes from an academic press, I'm on the receiving end of a flurry of emails and even some proposed edits to the first three chapters; I'm thrilled beyond belief, soaring high, ecstatic, telling all my friends and family, uncorking bottles of champagne. Then with no explanation whatsoever, I'm ghosted—literally—for eight months. I receive no response to my emails, phone calls. I even show up in person unannounced at the office and eventually crash a book launch party for a different memoir from the same publisher. Here I am, out at a bar with my friend Karin, *stalking* an editor and a fellow writer, buying a book I never intend to read and having the author sign it, just to get face time with these people and obtain the smallest hint of information about *my* book publication and where it's at. Still, it accomplishes nothing. I sink to a new all-time low.

I also find it interesting that the Christian book publishing world seems almost harder to break into than the traditional one. My writing definitely contains a faith element, with multiple references to scripture, my church, and so on. But this particular segment is dominated by only a few very selective publishing houses; for each of these, you must be *invited* to submit via contact with an agent or a professional editor. Or you can pay a substantial fee to upload your manuscript to an online Christian book portal that is reviewed by both agents and editors, and your book might even get a "gold, silver, or bronze" rating along with this, but no guarantees anyone would actually publish it. There are also self-publishing divisions of the larger companies that would be willing to publish (but only if it's under a certain word count and, again, for a large chunk of money) with the promise that if it starts to sell, it would get picked up by one of the Big Three—and I'm not talking about the Holy Trinity here. This almost seems more cutthroat than the secular equivalents; how un-Christian in my opinion. Isn't the entire point to share a story that might be salt and light potentially bringing others closer to God?

And that leads me to the vanity publishers, or the self-publishing route. So many companies are happy to take your money and print/publish your book for a hefty fee, but then what? What about editing, marketing, promotion, and so on?

The support seems lacking—unless, of course, you have a very thick wallet and could afford the "gold" or "platinum" package for extra services. I think of how valuable different voices can be in the fabric of the published literature, and I worry about how many people are excluded in the process if you must lay out that kind of money. Self-publishing is also a bit scary in the sense that if I get on a website and download an informational packet, this will often be followed by a barrage of high-pressure emails with pointed subject lines such as "We need to talk about your book" or "You must act now." Almost predatory in nature, these vanity publishers.

All the while, as part of my role in academic medicine, I am still composing and editing articles for potential publication in peer-reviewed journals—two parallel worlds in terms of my writing. But as I am doing this, I suddenly think, *Perhaps they can intersect?* Then I start to wonder, *Hey, maybe some of these very same journals will publish creative writing pieces written by a physician.*

I seek out submission categories such as "The Art of Medicine" or "On Being a Doctor" or "Perspectives." I spin off several book chapters and edit them to function as standalone essays. I first hear a yes from the *American Journal of Medicine*, then the *Journal of Clinical Oncology*, later *Annals of Family Medicine*—all fairly high-impact journals that apparently view my writing as worthy of publication. This is truly a shot in the arm, the much-needed confidence boost I've been seeking. I start to reason, *Hmm, I guess I could publish this book, just one chapter at a time.* It could take decades, eerily similar to how long it's taken me to get promoted.

Nevertheless, this positive experience gives me the courage to send the entire manuscript out again, which is critically important. If there is anything I've learned from the "ghosting" experience, it's to never assume anything without a book contract. On a writer's blog, I find a list of publishers that would accept online, un-agented submissions from first-time authors. Hooray! After paring down that list to about half (excluding children's books), I go to each of these websites, looking at the type of books they publish, what kind of authors, and so on, trying to find a good fit. This is a painstaking process, but very much worth the effort in the end.

As a matter of fact, after another two month wait, I hear a yes from a publisher in Chicago and another out of Oregon--in exactly the same week. At that point, with two affirmative responses on top of the initial interest from that academic press, I realize, *Wow, I think this dream is about to become a reality.*

I stop by a neighborhood liquor store on the way home and bought their most expensive bottle of pink champagne—I know, a bit trite. The label on this bottle of Moet & Chandon Rose Imperial even reminded me of the breast cancer ribbon. But later, having an actual signed contract in hand even long before the book was actually published opens many doors that I've never thought possible, including invitations to host book-signing parties, colleagues offering to leverage their connections for book reviews, even the medical school communications office reaching out to help publicize and promote the book and reach a wider audience.

I've once told a friend of mine that as a writer, having a book publication feels almost as significant as having a child. Her puzzled response is "But you're not a writer. You're a doctor." Okay, well, yes. I decide not to take offense at this comment. I guess it serves as a reminder that I probably shouldn't quit my day job. I even think back to the beginnings of my writing; once, I regretted the decision to take only two weeks off after surgery before I went back to work, because I could have requested much longer than that and devoted even more time to the book. But had I done that, I would not have experienced the patient encounters, the student teaching, the poignant interactions that immediately followed my return to work and served as inspiration for writing chapter after chapter. No, instead, doctoring and writing are *also* becoming inextricably linked in my world. I need to keep doing the former, to continue to excel at the latter.

There is actually a long history of physicians as writers, dating back to ancient times, the thought being that doctors are in a unique position to closely observe very dramatic moments of the human condition—birth, death, illness, and so on. Certainly, the intimate contact with patients and families, the full disclosure and exposure to all aspects of the physical and mental state would tend to inspire awe and creativity, or at the very least, wanting to record these stories for posterity's sake. And now, my experience of *physician as patient* truly adds to the mix. I also found so many instances of humor, irony, and downright ridiculousness within our health-care system; humor became a major coping mechanism for me and a great way to share potentially personal stories without creating too much tension or angst on the part of the listener.

So I decided to keep at it, keep submitting, keep writing, and see what happens. The biggest obstacle is carving out the time. I've become a bit of an insomniac as of late; early mornings over coffee becomes the perfect time to write—at my kitchen table, with a quiet house, and without competing activities. And I'm bringing my iPad with me everywhere, stashed in my purse, which helps immensely. I've edited chapters while sitting in the orthodontist's office, waiting for Sam to finish his appointment, or while watching Lydia's basketball practice. I've even edited using the Google Docs app on my phone while riding in the car across the state of South Dakota, traveling to a family reunion. Luckily, the keyboard Swype and the 5.5-inch display makes it feasible. And this is from someone who didn't own a smartphone until 2013, didn't start texting until 2015, and just engaged with social media in 2016.

And so, just as continuing to share patient stories would hopefully inspire other doctors to become better health-care providers, better patient advocates, and so on, perhaps sharing stories and observations about writing would inspire other budding authors to keep perfecting their craft.

To those of you already writing, I encourage you to keep at it! To others who only contemplate, well, if someone had told me what was going to happen in April 2016, all as a result of breast cancer—becoming a writer, getting a book published—I would have thought they were *insane.*

Never say never.

Chapter 25

TMI

There is no greater agony than bearing an untold story
inside you.
—Maya Angelou

Over time, I find myself struggling more and more with the
concept of oversharing, too much information, or "TMI"
—even after my colleague Dr. John Song told me it only
applies to surgeons. But still, I wonder if I am revealing too much
at times, having no filter, getting too personal—in particular when
it comes to my patients. In literature, physician self-disclosure has
been met with mixed results as to whether it benefits or detracts
from the doctor-patient relationship. And after all, isn't this the
opposite of what is generally taught in medical school? That in
order to maintain a professional working environment, we need
boundaries? We're told not to reveal too much about ourselves.
We don't want to compromise the doctor-patient relationship,
detract from the objectivity. Of course, a warm bedside manner is
helpful, but otherwise, keep the cards close to the chest.

But as I consider my own experience, I seem to have moved
in the opposite direction. And this started long before my
cancer diagnosis. I have been a primary care physician for over
sixteen years; along the way, I discovered that opening up to my
patients when asked or when the timing seemed right seemed to
strengthen the doctor-patient relationship. Sharing stories about

my family or my hobbies more quickly establishes rapport and a high level of trust than, say, discussing Minnesota weather. Becoming a mom in particular changed the dynamic with my mostly female panel; early on, we would commiserate about the tough stuff—breastfeeding woes, sleepless nights, *colic!*—while also sharing some mutually beneficial observations.

Then, of course, my perspective shifted even more starting in April 2016. Afterward, I was struck by how much more often breast cancer seemed to be showing up in my clinical practice. I opened up my schedule to new patients in 2017, one per clinic session, after reviewing the size of my panel and determining I had more capacity. At times, it seemed as though every new patient I met had a history of breast cancer or had just been diagnosed with breast cancer or was seeking treatment for recurrent or metastatic disease. I encountered many situations in which drawing upon my own experience would help the patient sitting right in front of me, and at times I had to ponder, *How much do I share?*

Adding to this dilemma is the fact that I chose to seek care within my own health system. As an unanticipated result, I'm getting many internal referrals—from my surgeon, his nurse, or my oncologist, her care team. If they see a patient with a new diagnosis of breast cancer who doesn't have a primary physician or needs a pre-op, guess who is next on their appointment list? I jokingly said at one point I should just relocate my practice to the second-floor Breast Center. That way, I can see patients right next to the key specialists involved in their care.

And I truly enjoy this newfound expertise, this connection, this synergy. I can relate to the fear and uncertainty immediately following a cancer diagnosis; not knowing the plan or the next steps until specific tests return certainly adds to the tension. Or feeling the need to clear various hurdles, such as pre-op chemotherapy prior to surgery or the multiple steps of reconstruction. So many psychological aspects are at play here, and they are often just as important as the physical ones.

I can also appreciate the controversies surrounding surgical decision-making, especially when it occurs at the height of a patient's anxiety. For instance, contralateral prophylactic mastectomy—having read about this extensively, even before consulting a surgeon, I soon realize there is no evidence for any cancer benefit using this approach. And yet, I recently had a healthy fifty-year-old patient of mine choose bilateral mastectomy with reconstruction for a tiny right-sided DCIS. While I supported her decision at every step of the way, a small part of me was cringing inside. She was clearly one of the most anxious patients I had ever met, regarding this diagnosis; her insistence of "Take them both off! Immediately!" I felt was directly related to her intense fear. She was also a non-English speaker; her daughter often interpreted for her. I could not help but wonder about informed decision-making, if there was any language barrier involved, and if she truly understood the major operation she was about to undertake for a lesion that is technically not considered "cancer" but rather a precancerous condition. There are even more recent studies suggesting it can be managed with medication, not surgery, with similar outcomes.

I also know in great detail the endocrine therapy and chemotherapy regimens typically offered to breast cancer patients, having been through this discussion myself. I have a heightened awareness of the side effects of tamoxifen after taking this drug for quite some time. I can share this knowledge with my patients, help inform the discussion; I find it extremely rewarding to be able to use my experience to help others. And I thought it might add to my credibility or strengthen the recommendations coming from oncology, maybe even lead to better outcomes by promoting patient adherence. I can say: "Just stay on tamoxifen for a while. The hot flashes should subside after a couple of months. Trust me, I've been there."

But it's hard, at times, to decide. Do I also tell this patient that I am a survivor myself? Or will that seem awkward, TMI? Or am I taking away from the conversation about them, just to describe my own journey? When deciding, I often try to pick up on certain cues, such as a patient being involved in an advocacy group. Or they have written something for a website or a blog or participated in a panel discussion, sharing their story with others; I reason they might appreciate more of the same. Or sometimes patients just point-blank ask me, "How do you know so much about breast cancer?"

At times, I choose to reveal this information; other times, not. But each instance that I have, surprisingly, patients have responded in an extremely positive fashion: thanking me for sharing, for opening up to them, shaking my hand, even giving me a hug. And for those internal referrals, I can relay the utmost confidence in their care team, because after all, I chose the same docs myself. All these have an incredible effect on relieving tension and stress. The very anxious patient I mentioned above? After I told her Dr. Anne Blaes was also my oncologist, that she's fantastic, and that I happen to know the field very well, she and her daughter visibly decompressed right in the exam room. The panic in their eyes dissipated, the furrowed brows relaxed, the clenched jaws eased into a slight smile. By the end of the visit, they both took turns shaking my hand, repeatedly expressing gratitude. I think about it from their perspective; if I were the patient, I would appreciate knowing my doctor has been through this too and understands my situation; it's an expression of empathy.

I sincerely hope that making these types of connections will benefit the patient in the long run. It might be even more significant for primary care since it could span many years and multiple health issues. Building trust becomes all the more important given the longitudinal nature of our working relationship. That's why I take the risk and open up in the first place. And recently, I inherited a patient where not only breast cancer but actually humor—mirth!—took center stage during our initial conversation.

I meet Erika as a new patient, my last one on a Tuesday afternoon. By midafternoon, the clinic's waiting areas are often somewhat crowded, and there may be a shortage of exam rooms, too, because schedules tend to run more and more behind as it gets later in the day. I was ready to see Erika at the designated appointment time, but I couldn't find a room or a rooming staff available to check her in. After scrolling through Epic a bit, I get up and start pacing around the collaboration zone, then out into the waiting area and back, then eventually I decide to step up and room the patient myself. I can see by the locator badge that she is sitting just outside the clinic entrance, but since this is my first time meeting her, I'm not exactly sure what she looks like or whom to approach. So I am forced to just step outside and call her name, "Erika?"

From behind me comes "I'm over here." I turn; I have walked right past her, in part because her hair is much shorter than the picture I see in Epic. Also, her eyes are closed in that photo—it was tough to get a visual for easy identification. I stop and smile, extend my hand, and say, "Pleased to meet you! Come back and follow me." She is frowning, maybe because the clinic is behind schedule or the lobby is too full or I had to call out her name to locate her—all of which has happened to me before, checking in on the second floor of the CSC. I can certainly relate.

We find an empty exam room, and I instruct her to take a seat next to the computer. I had reviewed her chart prior to this appointment, of course, and I found out that she is also a breast cancer survivor, diagnosed in 2011, stage III. She follows up with Dr. Douglas Yee, a university oncologist, who is also the director of the Masonic Cancer Center.

"Welcome to the PCC!" I say. "What brought you to clinic today?"

She still seems a tiny bit uncomfortable. "I am looking for another primary care physician. I was referred to a group near Stillwater. I live in Lake Elmo. But I just didn't really hit it off with the doctor there; I guess I didn't feel any connection. Plus, my oncologist, Dr. Yee, is here at the U. I thought it might be good to have everything in one place."

"Ah! That makes sense," I respond. I mention that Dr. Yee is top notch, a real pioneer in the field. I also say, "Well, you need to feel comfortable with your care team and the doctors involved in your treatment plan. That is important." I'm trying to start with open-ended questions and broad observations in hopes of getting to know her better and hearing more regarding her expectations and general preferences.

At this point, she warms up a bit, smiles, and says, "Some of this might be me as well. I tend to have a rather sarcastic sense of humor, an acerbic wit. Not everybody appreciates that."

Inwardly, I think, *Ah, now this might be the start of a great working relationship. Mirth is God's medicine!* I say, "Well, humor is an excellent coping mechanism. I would encourage that approach." Next is a standard opening line for me with new patients: "Tell me a bit about yourself and your overall health."

I learn that she works for the Minneapolis Police Department as an arson investigator. How interesting. She goes on to outline the details surrounding her breast cancer treatment, including bilateral mastectomy, followed by chemotherapy, radiation, and later endocrine therapy. I congratulate her on being seven years out from all this.

All the while, I am picking up on the fact that, indeed, she *does* have a wicked sense of humor. Erika describes hosting a "burn the bra" party after her mastectomy operation, even goes into detail about the remnants of the bonfire in her backyard the next day, including all the leftover underwire. She also mentions being a writer herself in that she sent a monthly newsletter to all her friends and family to keep them posted throughout her cancer journey, sprinkled with funny anecdotes. In her line of work, she also describes how gallows humor and even practical jokes from coworkers in the police force helped her cope, keep her sanity, and stay positive despite the situation.

At this point, listening intently, I feel led to open up to Erika; I had a hunch that this might help ease her mind when it comes to establishing rapport with a new primary care doctor. "I am a breast cancer survivor myself, two years out. In fact, you and I had the same surgeon, Dr. Todd Tuttle. And now I can see he was a good fit for you too. He has a keen sense of humor!"

"Really? That's great!" she says and agrees with me. "I even pulled a prank on Dr. Tuttle on the day of surgery."

I smile and say, "Please tell me more."

"You know how surgeons have the safety maneuver, marking the site of the operation on the patient's body? I decided to show up that morning with something else written on my chest, under the gown, in indelible ink: *'Used bumpers for sale, $200 or best offer.'*"

I laugh out loud and applaud her bravery. "You probably made his day!" I went on to describe how I also tried to joke around with Dr. Tuttle on the morning of my operation, saying when he walked into the room, "Boy, am I glad to see you. I have something to get off my chest!"

Now, we are both cracking up and enjoying the newfound connection. And I'm honestly thinking, *This can't be random—the fact that Erika happened to land on my schedule that afternoon out of a list of over twenty primary care doctors in the PCC.* Maybe Dr. Yee steered her in my direction, or perhaps it is providence. But I am looking forward to getting to know Erika, not just the health issues but also to hear more of her stories.

The importance of hearing a patient's narrative, not just medical but personal as well, it is incredibly beneficial in the long run. As an aside, it's also probably why I tend to run days behind in terms of Epic tasks. I don't like logging in to the computer while in the exam room, at least not until the very end; it detracts from the connection and my ability to listen and observe. I'd rather be fully present in the moment. But as a result, I often have to catch up in the evenings and on weekends to finish notes or whittle down the in-basket. For me, it's a small price to pay, though, because of exactly this type of interaction; the reward is huge. It's honestly why I went into medicine in the first place.

We go back to discussing Erika's more recent health; I ask how she is tolerating the aromatase inhibitor. "I still have occasional hot flashes, but not as severe as before." Erika has lymphedema of the left arm but manages well with regular massage therapy and Kinesio tape. She also reports mild numbness in her feet, a residual effect of chemotherapy. Despite all this, she exercises five times a week and remains very active; I encourage her to continue doing that. We'll also keep an eye on her blood pressure, I mention, which has been borderline at a few clinic visits.

At the conclusion of the appointment, Erika shakes my hand and even says, "I'm sorry if I seemed grouchy at the beginning of this visit."

I reassure her and mention that the first encounter at any clinic isn't easy and our tech-driven building makes it even harder, in some ways. I reply, "I think this is the start of a great working relationship."

After, I was very grateful for the opportunity to have this conversation. I would reflect once again on the fine line between TMI and connecting on a deeper level. I have no easy answers, here; I'm still trying to navigate every individual patient encounter, each unique situation. But some very positive things have come about as a result of opening up.

And maybe there is just something about breast cancer, too; perhaps the same principles would not apply if it were colon cancer or heart disease or diabetes. Breast cancer itself can be an affront not just to overall health but to femininity, body image, sexual well-being, and so on; because of that, those who survive it might feel a unique bond, a sisterhood of sorts thereafter.

That sisterhood is also extremely large and growing, given how common the disease, and that survivorship thankfully is increasing. And since this is almost exclusively a women's health issue, women might feel more compelled to support one another through it and more empowered to bond over it—and hopefully through more than just wearing a pink ribbon.

Making personal connections, allowing authenticity and vulnerability to permeate relationships, I believe can only serve to strengthen them. Ultimately, that is a large part of what gives survivors the courage to keep fighting—to know that others have been there, too, and are fighting alongside them. For all this and more, I see many potential benefits to sharing stories and will continue to do so.

Yes, even ones that might approach TMI.

Chapter 26

WELCOME TO THE CLUB

God, your love came crashing in, and pulled me out of
the fire; I'm a survivor.
—Zach Williams

My one-year follow-up with Dr. Anne Blaes finally
occurs. And thankfully, the disturbing dreams I have
leading up to it are just that—nightmares, not reality.

Right before the appointment, I have a left-sided 3-D
mammogram that is immediately read as negative, bringing a
huge sigh of relief. I'm so grateful that the breast center radiologists
interpret the scan right there on the spot; I am sure they appreciate
the fact that waiting, for any length of time, will be torture for a
cancer survivor.

As I am being checked in, I note my blood pressure reading
is completely normal. My weight is also back up, approaching
the same number I saw on the scale all through my twenties and
early thirties—before kids, of course—what I would consider my
"fighting weight." I am escorted back to an exam room; after a
short wait and a knock, in walks Dr. Anne Blaes.

"Hi there! How have you been?"

I tell her, "Great! Feeling really good!"

We both share the good news of the negative mammogram,
normal blood pressure, gaining back some of the weight I lost.
I also describe my ongoing commitment to exercise, just having

completed my very first indoor triathlon at the University Rec Center, the Tri-U-Mah.

"So," she says, "no lingering effects from the axillary web syndrome?" I tell her no, that it never recurred, and that I'm back to full range of motion, which was especially important for the swim portion of the event. Next, she asks how I was tolerating tamoxifen.

I tell Anne, "It's my new favorite drug. I'm having zero side effects, the hot flashes are gone, my weight has stabilized, and personally, I'm thrilled to not have a period anymore! I'll stay on it for the rest of my life!"

She laughs then goes on to confirm a completely normal physical exam and recommends some routine tests, such as a cholesterol panel and a bone density scan, at a future date. It's a great visit—boring, almost, but in a very good way.

What I really notice about the appointment, however, this time around, has nothing to do with me, my health, nor the tablet check-in, the locator badge, the technician, the radiologist, the rooming staff, the nurses, or even the doctors. All around the Breast Center and the Masonic Cancer Center, second floor of the CSC, several interactions occur that make me feel as though I have been indoctrinated into an exclusive club.

Prior to the mammogram, I take a seat next to an older lady with curly gray hair just outside the radiology suite; she glances over at me, smiles, and says, "I am a breast cancer survivor, three years out! How about you?"

To this, I reply, "It's my one-year cancer-versary."

"Congratulations!" she said. "Love that term!"

I tell her at our house my nine-year-old daughter came up with it, and she proceeds to show me pictures of her grandkids on her phone. Sitting right across from us is a middle-aged man; he comments, "Good job, you two! I'm five years out, and doing great!"

I am reminded at that moment in time that, yes, men can get breast cancer too.

The very same thing occurs in the waiting area outside Clinic 2B. There is a rather young-appearing woman sitting next to her husband across from me on a loveseat, a low coffee table between us. They are chatting about her upcoming appointment.

She then turns to me and says, "Are you here to see Dr. Blaes, too? We just love her!"

And then: I see one of my patients, whom I know quite well, strolling through the lobby. I wave, and smile; she quickly strides over to me, as I am standing up from my chair, upon hearing a nurse call my name to bring me back. She extends her hand, saying, "Dr. Thompson! It's so good to see you!" I shake her hand and say hello but then the nurse is calling my name again. As I turn to leave, I hear her say to another patient waiting in the lobby: "That's my primary care doctor! She's great!"

The other patient replies: "What is she doing *here*?"

On and on it went. I notice it more than ever before, for some reason. I saw perfect strangers sharing stories about their health, their lives, their last PET CT result, even horror stories about chemo or radiation—all supporting one another throughout the process in their own unique way.

I'm struck by this fact, thinking, Wow, this is the polar opposite of what hospital attorneys and HIPAA would make us believe—that privacy is valued at all costs, over and above what benefit there might be in sharing, spontaneously opening up to others in the most unlikely of situations.

Maybe, just maybe, I've gotten it all wrong about the new clinic building. Perhaps the open-lobby concept, the shared workstations, the collaboration zones, the touchdown spaces could all be viewed as a way to facilitate more personal contact, more face time, more verbal communication, more interactions. And not just individually or one-on-one, such as doctor and patient, but by groups of people, across professions, across disciplines, including what I just observed that day. This open floor plan brings patients and families in closer proximity to one another while waiting for a lab draw, an X-ray, or an appointment. It's not necessarily a design flaw or to save square footage but intentional, to underscore the point that we're all in this together.

Thinking more about this, I recall my patient Laurie and the poem she had sent to me; after checking out, I take a seat in the waiting area, pull up her email on my phone, and reread the final lines.

> You have joined the millions of
> others, you have CANCER.
> It changes your life. Whether
> contained or not you can never go
> back.
> Survivors are who we are.
> We are in an exclusive club that no
> one wants to join. But once we join,
> we feel an instant bond with all the
> other people who have been given
> that horrible one-word diagnosis.
> I did not understand this before,
> but now that I have joined the club,
> I get it.
> Survivors see the world just a little
> bit differently. (Laurie Azine)

Indeed, an instant bond, an exclusive club.

Right then and there, at that particular moment in time, I thought, *I get it, too.*

Chapter 27

THE JOURNEY AHEAD: ENJOY THE RIDE

If you've been walking the same old road for miles and miles,
If you've been hearing the same old voice tell the same old lies,
If you're trying to fill the same old holes inside,
there's a better life . . .
—Zach Williams

These just happen to be two favorite songs of mine, "Chainbreaker" and "Survivor," both by Christian artist Zach Williams.

Also, "Chainbreaker" is the title and theme of a long-distance cycling event, the Chainbreaker Ride. This annual fundraiser benefits cancer research at the University of Minnesota, and I was able to participate in 2017 and 2018.

As time marches on, I've been thinking a lot about that word, *survivor*. Many patients and friends of mine who have been treated for cancer do not like the term, even shy away from it. Some feel it is overused or abused as a rallying cry of sorts, for many different purposes, legitimate or not. Others would rather not be labeled, compartmentalized, defined by a disease, or they simply might not want to draw attention to the fact that they are a survivor, while others are not. However, I found the National Cancer Institute has a clear definition: "An individual is considered a cancer survivor from the time of diagnosis through the balance of his or her life." The oncology field obviously needs terminology when studying patient outcomes, preventing recurrence, reducing long-term complications, and extending life. At the end of the day, we have to call ourselves *something*, I guess.

Less than twelve months out from my own diagnosis, I was intrigued to receive an email in February 2017 from the dean, describing the Chainbreaker as an event to bring together the university community and to support the Masonic Cancer Center. My resident in clinic at the time, Nick, also read it and commented that his medical school hosts a similar annual event called the Pelotonia, which began in 2008 and has raised over $184 million to date for cancer research.

Wow, I thought, *that's kind of a big deal.* Maybe I should show support for my fellow survivors, my home institution, my own treatment team, and sign up for this. Also, in recent years, I had been getting back into bicycling once again.

This was a big part of my life in junior high, riding my bike all summer long, day in, day out, usually with my good friend Laurie, who lived mere blocks from me. In the town of Milaca, I would ride for hours my stylin' blue Huffy ten-speed that was purchased at the local Hardware Hank. No helmet, bike jersey, bike shorts, or clip-ins, just daisy duke cutoffs, Ocean Pacific T-shirts, Nike tennis shoes. And no bike lock either—we would simply prop up the bikes against the brick wall of the Dairy Queen if we wanted to go in for a soft serve cone. Laurie and I would disappear for the entire day, dawn till dusk, other than to pop back into my house or her grandma's for a meal or a snack. Mom never even knew where I was at any given time; we could be down by the Rum River, riding our bikes along the trails, where we stopped to wade in the water, or out on the country roads on the outskirts of town.

Ah, to grow up in a small town in Minnesota in the eighties; my kids hear these stories and are insanely jealous of the freedoms we had—although, I have to say, the single biggest scar I have on my body (until recently) is on my right knee, and it is from biking. Laurie and I once got caught up in each other's paths coming down a steep hill and wiped out, resulting in both of us landing on the pavement with my right leg covered in road rash and a deep divot on the side of my knee. It's still visible to this day, but it's almost a source of pride. I shared this story with Lydia once after a tree branch took her down while biking on the Lake Como path and also told it to Sam upon seeing him launch over his handlebars due to hitting a pothole. No pain, no gain.

Three summers before the Chainbreaker, my segue back into biking was jump-started by an impulse buy while visiting Milaca; at a local thrift store, there sat a powder-blue and yellow Schwinn World Sport women's ten-speed, so very similar to my bike from the eighties, truly vintage but in great shape. It appeared barely ridden. For $25, I took it home in the back of my Durango and rode that tank for two seasons before investing another dime in it. This was also something I could do with Sam and Lydia; riding our bikes around Lake Como in St. Paul with the obligatory stop for ice cream at the Pavilion is an outing we could all enjoy. And while flying down the hill on Lexington Parkway, wind in my hair, sitting back and letting gravity do all the work, hearing that familiar *tick, tick, tick* sound from the bike, I truly felt like a teenager again. Eventually, I did invest in a bike helmet after hearing so much flak from my kids when not wearing one.

So upon hearing about the Chainbreaker, with the inaugural ride happening in August of 2017, I took the plunge and signed up immediately. Too soon, actually; I paid a $99 registration fee that later was waived to attract more participants. But over one thousand riders registered, and the spring before, I dusted off the Schwinn and even took it to my neighborhood bike shop for a tune-up and new tires. This also gave me the motivation to bike longer distances to train for the fifty-mile ride; my good friend Karin and I would meet up on the weekends and bike twenty miles or so. She introduced me to several bike trails and paths around the Twin Cities, including the Gateway, the Greenway, and along the River Road, with a stop at Sea Salt. I even started biking to work, finding a route that was almost completely protected from traffic via the Transit Way.

And this was all very enjoyable, not just the bike rides, but the other Chainbreaker events leading up to it, such as the kickoff party at Surly or the Fulton Brewery outing, known as Chainbreaker on Deck. At these events, I would mingle with many colleagues from the U, some of whom I found out were cancer survivors themselves or had a spouse or a family member affected by the disease. Several in attendance obviously knew why I was there, but many did not.

Eventually, by midsummer, I decided to purchase a new bike that would make the long distance rides more comfortable; I saved up some moonlighting money and would give my old Schwinn to Lydia. This was actually quite a process; I researched carbon frame road bikes extensively online, read reviews, then drove to just about every Erik's in the Twin Cities for test rides before finally settling on a 2015 Raleigh Capri. It's turquoise blue with accents of pink, and compared to the World Sport, it is lightning fast—so much that I nicknamed it the Flash. And it also happened that my kid's favorite superhero show at the time was *The Flash*. It fit perfectly.

Our Division of General Internal Medicine, on Brad Benson's suggestion, formed a team, or a peloton, for the Chainbreaker. It's a way to share fundraising support, but it also boosts morale and promotes team building and camaraderie. Mike Rhodes even designed a very stylish bike jersey for us all to wear, sporting the maroon and gold colors. Even more poignant was the fact that several of our gen med faculty members were in the midst of battling cancer themselves; John Song was still facing multiple rounds of preoperative chemotherapy for pancreatic cancer, Charlie Moldow had just completed radiation for Merkel cell carcinoma, Wes Miller was recently diagnosed with esophageal cancer. Our peloton's name, GIM Band, had this tagline: "We're riding with a Song in our hearts."

Another truly moving event for me was the Friday night opening ceremony. Great food, live music, and inspirational stories from supporters—I found this touching and so very humbling to see some riders there who had even lost a limb to sarcoma and were still going the distance. I had a few moments where I choked up and fought back tears that evening, thinking, *I am so blessed to be healthy enough to do something this physically active, biking fifty miles to benefit cancer research, just one year after the entire ordeal.* I also had the idea to invite Karin along to the opening ceremony, to use my extra ticket; she was a cyclist, so I knew she'd enjoy the event. And I wanted to thank her as the very first donor on my website and taking extra time to train me in on the long-distance rides.

Then comes the actual day of the Chainbreaker, the ride itself. I set my phone alarm for 5:00 a.m. to leave the house by 6:00; I'm woken up out of a very vivid dream and with the need to get out there so early and the overall anticipation and the adrenaline rush. All together I'm feeling kind of stressed, anxious for some odd reason. Even though I know the ride, the route, and that the weather forecast is fabulous, still I have a lot of nervous energy. Or maybe it's just the cup of coffee followed by the Diet Mountain Dew in the car.

I drive to the starting point in Eagan, park, get out, then head over to the bike corral to pick up the Flash. It's about 6:20 a.m., and although it's early, I am truly grateful for the morning start, knowing we would escape any heat later in the day. After I get my bike, I wait for a couple more minutes. Then I spot Todd Tuttle in the same parking lot with his Bianchi in that instantly recognizable color known as celeste. I walk over with a big smile, and we greet each other. Then we head over to the picnic area to get snacks and top off our water bottles. In just a few more minutes, we are already being asked to line up at the starting point; three of the GIM Band peloton are in the middle of the pack of fifty-mile riders. And at 7:00 a.m., the ride begins.

I find my resident Nick Zorko, and we fall into stride very quickly. Our pace is quite evenly matched. Side by side, or single file, we are averaging about seventeen miles per hour, and this feels perfect to me, not to slow, not too fast, just right. After getting out of the city, we take in the lovely views of the countryside: the rolling hills, the fields of corn, cattle grazing, horses trotting through a pasture. It's a perfect sunny morning and not too hot. No rain, thank goodness. Later, the route circles beside a lake, and the last twelve miles are mostly downhill on a shady tree-lined trail along the beautiful Cannon River. Seeing boats out on the water or canoes and kayaks on the river reminds me of Lake Mille Lacs—an idyllic picture of summer in Minnesota.

And for the entire ride, almost four hours, I get the opportunity to engage with multiple colleagues, share stories along the way. I jokingly say it's much easier to ride with a bunch of guys than with Karin, because she and I tend to talk *so* much. We'll get short of breath climbing a steep hill. I get to know Nick, hearing about his hometown in Ohio, his current research interests, his future plans in oncology. I bike some of the stretch with Bill Conroy; we chat about the PCC and plans for the Signature Health program but also discuss riding a bike growing up. The second twenty-five miles, I ride alongside Todd Tuttle, and when biking through a few small towns, I mention how similar they are to Milaca. He also turns out to be perfect for drafting when I need a break from the wind resistance. But mostly, I just enjoy the company, the perfect bike ride on a lovely summer day, the bonding, creating shared memories. And all for such a great cause—that's very significant to me. And it reminds me of the importance of team in every sense of the word. No matter what happens down the road in terms of my health, I want to enjoy the ride, and I'm so grateful to know I can lean on my colleagues when I need support. And I am reminded of how much more you can accomplish—how much farther you can ride—when in a group, as opposed to an individual effort.

The finish line celebration is another memorable part of this day. First is the massage tent—a perfect ending, working out those sore spots in my shoulders from holding position on the bike. Then the food—it's quite a spread, almost everything under the sun. There are chicken fajitas and burgers for the meat lovers, black bean quinoa and other green salads for the health nuts, assorted chips, and side dishes. There's even a vast array of cake pops for dessert, in case the samples from Vice Cream with naughty names, such as Afternoon Delight, don't provide enough satisfaction for the sweet tooth. Lots of people are gathered under the big tent, including many friends and colleagues I know well, such as seeing Anne Blaes and her staff at one of the tables and chatting with them for a bit. It's a lively group. It feels like a real party; the beer tent even serves one of my favorite IPAs, Fulton Sweet Child of Vine, and the entertainment includes live music from GB Leighton. The entire atmosphere feels almost like a German Oktoberfest kind of celebration, only without the lederhosen.

The night before, the riders were asked to write on a display board whom they were riding for. I tried to ponder those in my life who were battling cancer: Charles Moldow, Wes Miller, and John Song again came to mind, as three colleagues and mentors in the Department of Medicine. I don't have anyone in my family with this disease, and so I wrote their names on the board. That same board was transported to the fifty-mile finish line celebration, and that afternoon, I read through the names and heartwarming inscriptions with interest.

Then, while doing that, I remembered, *Wait, I am a breast cancer survivor too!* Honestly, at times I feel so good and so healthy I sometimes forget that ever happened. Or perhaps there is a part of me that *wants* to forget about it. Still, I didn't think to write my own name despite collecting two jersey badges at the event: "Survivor" and "Living Proof."

Instead, I'll just keep it written in my mind or in this chapter—that beautiful day, the significance behind it, the many reasons why I ride, even the meaning behind the name of the event: Chainbreaker . . . By the grace of God, I feel I have broken free of multiple chains in my life. And that tune by Zach Williams I will play on Spotify over and again—so inspiring.

> *If you've got pain, He's a pain taker.*
> *If you feel lost, He's a way maker.*
> *If you need freedom, or saving, He's a*
> *prison shaking savior;*
> *If you've got chains, He's a Chainbreaker.*

I might even be up for a Chainbreaker part III.

About the Author

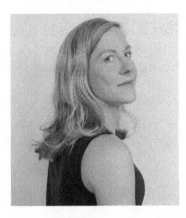

Dr. Heather Thompson Buum is an assistant professor at the University of Minnesota in the Division of General Internal Medicine. She graduated from Hamline University in 1993 with a BA in biology, then went on to complete both medical school and residency at the University of Minnesota. She joined the faculty in 2002 and devotes half her time to patient care, practicing both outpatient primary care and inpatient hospital medicine. The remaining time, she spends in various teaching and administrative roles. She formerly served as an associate program director for the internal medicine residency and now is a course director for Human Health and Disease and a small group facilitator for Essentials of Clinical Medicine in the medical school. Dr. Thompson has won numerous awards for both teaching and patient care, including Outstanding Medical School Teacher in 2016, the Department of Medicine Clinical Excellence Award in 2013, and *Minnesota Monthly*'s Top Doctors for Women in 2013 and 2011. She is a member of the Society for General Internal Medicine and a fellow in the American College of Physicians. Her outside interests include choral music, performing with the Oratorio Society of Minnesota for over twenty years. She also enjoys cooking, running, and an occasional round of golf. She lives with her husband and two children in St. Paul.

CREDITS

Mirth is God's Medicine

- The Chapter "Breaking Bad, Part II' was first published as the essay "Out of the Mouths of Babes" in category The Art of Oncology in the *Journal of Clinical Oncology*, November 2018.

- The Chapter "You've Got Mail" will be published as an essay in the category of Healing Arts, *Journal of General Internal Medicine*, August 2019.

With Mirth and Laughter

- The Chapter "TMI" was first published as "Sharing My Diagnosis: How Much is Too Much?" in the *Annals of Family Medicine*, March 2019.

- The Chapter "My Love/Hate Relationship with Technology" was first published as "See One, Be One, Teach One: How Becoming a Patient informed my role as a Teaching Physician" in the *American Journal of Medicine*, February 2019.

- The poem by Laurie Azine referenced in Chapter 2 was first published as "Medicine from the Other Side of the Tracks" in *Minnesota Medicine*, September 2010.

ACKNOWLEDGMENTS

My second book was released so soon after the first that I contemplated using the very same acknowledgments page for both. Then, I thought the better of it, realizing this was an opportunity to thank new people who had come alongside me in the process, as well as the same group of supportive friends, family, church family, and colleagues mentioned before.

I have often said in those "elevator conversations" that book 1 is about doctor as patient, while book 2 is about patient as doctor—two halves of the same story. I really enjoyed writing book 2 because it is less about me and more about my patients, friends, family, students, and residents—a rich tapestry of stories that illustrate the humanity of us all—and about how being in this dual role of doctor and patient continues to teach me more helpful life lessons.

So first and foremost, I'd like to thank my patients, especially those who graciously allowed me to share their personal story in print, giving me permission to write about them in a format for potentially all the world to read. Your openness and willingness to share, I know, will benefit many other patients, families, doctors, caregivers, and teachers.

Of course, I need to again thank my family—Paul, Sam, and Lydia—for their support and also their patience, as getting two books ready for publication in a span of a few months took much of my time and energy and monopolized every dinner conversation for a period of time. They understood how big this was for me, and their excitement and enthusiasm helped keep me going even when I had my own doubts and fears that I could pull this off.

I would also like to thank my publisher, John Paul Owles, for taking a chance on me and taking the time to read not one but two book manuscripts and agreeing to publish both. And this is without insisting on a specific word count or asking me to condense the two into one, as other publishers seemed wont to do. I truly believe the final product is much better, and not just having two sides of the same story but being able to keep all the influential parts of both. Hopefully, it will reach a wider audience and benefit more people in the process.

Dr. Jon Hallberg deserves special thanks as a colleague who immediately came alongside me when he heard of my upcoming book publication, offering to assist with specific reviews and publicity, as well as hosting a book launch party at his beautiful Mill City Clinic. His support of the arts and humanities in medicine truly makes the Twin Cities and the University of Minnesota Medical School a much better place to live, teach, and practice.

Finally, all the glory goes to God, who sustained me through this entire ordeal and somehow gifted me with writing in the midst of it. Experiencing the therapeutic aspects of writing and the power of narrative medicine has been life-changing for me; I look forward to many more years, God willing, of being able to continue doing it. Theologian John Piper once wrote a book entitled *Don't Waste Your Cancer.* I wholeheartedly embrace this philosophy, and I believe writing helps me accomplish just that. Whatever comes my way, no matter what the future may hold, I will remain open to receiving it, learning from it, and using it to help others, trusting that He has a plan. And to cancer, I will simply quote scripture and say this:

You intended to harm me, but God intended it for good
to accomplish what is now being done,
the saving of many lives.
Genesis 50:20

MIRTH IN MEDICINE SERIES

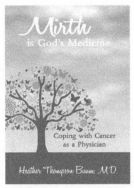

"*Mirth is God's Medicine* is the story of a wife, a mother, and a physician stepping into the shoes of a patient. It is not only informative, but it is full of valuable insight and observations for doctors, nurses, and other clinicians, as well as medical students and residents, direct from one of their own." —Margaret Lesh, Author of *Let Me Get This Off My Chest: A Breast Cancer Survivor Over-Shares.*

As a primary care physician in her mid-forties, Dr. Heather Thompson is diagnosed with breast cancer; she is now facing multiple medical decisions, this time about her own health. Experiencing the system firsthand informs her future approach in unanticipated ways; what initially seems like a negative event becomes a process of growth and transformation. The story illustrates how a doctor, as both informed medical professional and human being, copes with a new diagnosis and disease.

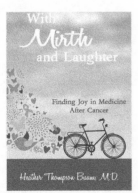

With Mirth and Laughter moves beyond the early days of Dr. Thompson's breast cancer treatment, including surgery, medication, and physical therapy, and further describes how a cancer diagnosis impacts her friendships, family dynamics, teaching and mentoring roles. More importantly, it changes her practice style and view of what it means to provide patient centered care. This book includes story after story of patient interactions, some ironic, many humorous, but all poignant and compelling; they serve to illustrate how being in one role ultimately benefits the other. Dr. Thompson also chronicles how becoming a patient changes her approach in how she teaches and trains future physicians. Those in academic medicine or in a teaching role of any kind can relate.